Emergency and Critical Care

Editors

VANESSA L. COOK
DIANA M. HASSEL

VETERINARY CLINICS OF NORTH AMERICA: EQUINE PRACTICE

www.vetequine.theclinics.com

Consulting Editor
A. SIMON TURNER

August 2014 • Volume 30 • Number 2

ELSEVIER

1600 John F. Kennedy Boulevard • Suite 1800 • Philadelphia, Pennsylvania, 19103-2899

http://www.vetequine.theclinics.com

VETERINARY CLINICS OF NORTH AMERICA: EQUINE PRACTICE Volume 30, Number 2
August 2014 ISSN 0749-0739, ISBN-13: 978-0-323-32028-3

Editor: Patrick Manley
Developmental Editor: Donald Mumford

Veterinary Clinics of North America: Equine Practice (ISSN 0749-0739) is published in April, August, and December by Elsevier Inc., 360 Park Avenue South, New York, NY 10010-1710. Business and Editorial Offices: 1600 John F. Kennedy Blvd., Suite 1800, Philadelphia, PA 19103-2899. Subscription prices are $270.00 per year (domestic individuals), $431.00 per year (domestic institutions), $130.00 per year (domestic students/residents), $315.00 per year (Canadian individuals), $543.00 per year (Canadian institutions), $365.00 per year (international individuals), $543.00 per year (international institutions), and $180.00 per year (international and Canadian students/residents). To receive student/resident rate, orders must be accompanied by name of affiliated institution, date of term, and the signature of program/residency coordinator on institution letterhead. Orders will be billed at individual rate until proof of status is received. Foreign air speed delivery is included in all *Clinics* subscription prices. All prices are subject to change without notice. **POSTMASTER:** Send address changes to *Veterinary Clinics of North America: Equine Practice*, 3251 Riverport Lane, Maryland Heights, MO 63043. Customer Service (orders, claims, online, change of address): Elsevier Health Sciences Division, Subscription Customer Service, 3251 Riverport Lane, Maryland Heights, MO 63043. Tel: 1-800-654-2452 (U.S. and Canada); 314-447-8871 (outside U.S. and Canada). Fax: 314-447-8029. E-mail: journalscustomerservice-usa@elsevier.com (for print support); E-mail: journalsonlinesupport-usa@elsevier.com (for online support).

Reprints. For copies of 100 or more of articles in this publication, please contact the Commercial Reprints Department, Elsevier Inc., 360 Park Avenue South, New York, NY 10010-1710. Tel.: 212-633-3874; Fax: 212-633-3820; E-mail: reprints@elsevier.com.

Veterinary Clinics of North America: Equine Practice is covered in *MEDLINE/PubMed (Index Medicus)*, *Excerpta Medica, Current Contents/Agriculture, Biology and Environmental Sciences*, and *ISI*.

Contributors

CONSULTING EDITOR

A. SIMON TURNER, BVSc, MS, DVSc
Diplomate, American College of Veterinary Surgeons; Professor Emeritus, Department of Clinical Sciences, College of Veterinary Medicine and Biomedical Sciences, Colorado State University, Fort Collins, Colorado

EDITORS

VANESSA L. COOK, VetMB, PhD
Diplomate, American College of Veterinary Surgeons; Diplomate, American College of Veterinary Emergency and Critical Care; Associate Professor, Department of Large Animal Clinical Sciences, Michigan State University College of Veterinary Medicine, East Lansing, Michigan

DIANA M. HASSEL, DVM, PhD
Diplomate, American College of Veterinary Surgeons; Diplomate, American College of Veterinary Emergency and Critical Care; Associate Professor, Department of Clinical Sciences, College of Veterinary Medicine and Biological Sciences, Colorado State University, Fort Collins, Colorado

AUTHORS

BRANDY A. BURGESS, DVM, MSc, PhD
Diplomate of American College of Veterinary Internal Medicine (Large Animal); Department of Population Health Sciences, Virginia-Maryland Regional College of Veterinary Medicine, Virginia Tech, Blacksburg, Virginia

ELIZABETH A. CARR, DVM, PhD
Diplomate of American College of Veterinary Internal Medicine; Diplomate of American College of Veterinary Emergency and Critical Care Medicine; Associate Professor, Department of Large Animal Clinical Sciences, College of Veterinary Medicine, Michigan State University, East Lansing, Michigan

VANESSA L. COOK, VetMB, PhD
Diplomate, American College of Veterinary Surgeons; Diplomate, American College of Veterinary Emergency and Critical Care; Associate Professor, Department of Large Animal Clinical Sciences, Michigan State University College of Veterinary Medicine, East Lansing, Michigan

KEVIN THOMAS TRENT CORLEY, BVM&S, PhD, MRCVS
Diplomate, American College of Veterinary Internal Medicine; Diplomate, American College of Veterinary Emergency and Critical Care; Diplomate, European College of Equine Internal Medicine; Veterinary Advances Ltd, Co Kildare, Ireland

KIRA L. EPSTEIN, DVM
Diplomate, American College of Veterinary Surgeons; Diplomate, American College of Veterinary Emergency and Critical care; Clinical Associate Professor, Department of Large Animal Medicine, College of Veterinary Medicine, University of Georgia, Athens, Georgia

LANGDON FIELDING, DVM
Diplomate, American College of Veterinary Emergency and Critical Care; Loomis Basin Equine Medical Center, Penryn, California

R. REID HANSON, DVM
Diplomate, American College of Veterinary Surgeons; Diplomate, American College of Veterinary Emergency and Critical care; Professor, Auburn University College of Veterinary Medicine, Auburn, Alabama

DIANA M. HASSEL, DVM, PhD
Diplomate, American College of Veterinary Surgeons; Diplomate, American College of Veterinary Emergency and Critical Care; Associate Professor, Department of Clinical Sciences, College of Veterinary Medicine and Biological Sciences, Colorado State University, Fort Collins, Colorado

JONNA MAARIA JOKISALO, DVM
Diplomate, American College of Veterinary Internal Medicine; Chief of Emergency and Critical Care Medicine, Animagi Hevossairaala Hyvinkää, Hyvinkää, Finland

SARAH LE JEUNE, DVM
Diplomate, American College of Veterinary Surgeons; Diplomate, American College of Veterinary Sports Medicine and Rehabilitation; Department of Surgical and Radiological Sciences, University of California, Davis, California

JAMES N. MOORE, DVM, PhD
Distinguished Research Professor, Departments of Large Animal Medicine, and Physiology and Pharmacology, College of Veterinary Medicine, University of Georgia, Athens, Georgia

PAUL S. MORLEY, DVM, PhD
Diplomate of American College of Veterinary Internal Medicine (Large Animal); Department of Clinical Sciences, James L. Voss Veterinary Teaching Hospital, Colorado State University, Fort Collins, Colorado

MARGARET C. MUDGE, VMD
Associate Professor, Department of Veterinary Clinical Sciences, The Ohio State University, Columbus, Ohio

AMELIA S. MUNSTERMAN, DVM, MS
Diplomate, American College of Veterinary Surgeons; Diplomate, American College of Veterinary Emergency and Critical care; Clinical Lecturer, Auburn University College of Veterinary Medicine, Auburn, Alabama

JON PALMER, VMD
Diplomate American College of Veterinary Internal Medicine, Director of Perinatology/Neonatology Programs; Chief, Neonatal Intensive Care Service, Graham French Neonatal Section, Connelly Intensive Care Unit, New Bolton Center, University of Pennsylvania

BRETT TENNENT-BROWN, BVSc, MS
Diplomate American College of Veterinary Internal Medicine; Diplomate American College of Veterinary Emergency and Critical Care; Senior Lecturer in Equine Medicine; Faculty of Veterinary Science, Equine Centre, The University of Melbourne, Werribee, Victoria, Australia

MICHEL L. VANDENPLAS, PhD
Senior Scientist, Ross University School of Veterinary Medicine, Basseterre, Saint Kitts, West Indies

MARY BETH WHITCOMB, DVM, MBA
Department of Surgical and Radiological Sciences, University of California, Davis, California

Contents

The purpose of this article is to provide a quick reference for field triage of the sick neonatal foal. Therefore, information is focused toward diagnostics and treatments that can be performed in the field. When evaluating a weak, recumbent, or lethargic foal on a farm, it is often difficult to make a definitive diagnosis. Therefore, the approach should be to treat what is treatable and prevent what is preventable. In many cases, the goal will be to stabilize a foal before referral to a tertiary care facility where more intensive and continuous treatment can be performed.

RECOVER was created to optimize survival of small animal patients from cardiopulmonary arrest. Several findings from this study are applicable to cardiopulmonary resuscitation in the neonatal foal. In particular, chest compressions should be a priority with no pauses and a "push hard, push fast" approach. The importance of ventilation is minimized with short, infrequent breaths at a rate of 10 to 20 per minute recommended.

Despite advances in neonatal intensive care sepsis, severe sepsis and septic shock remain the biggest killers of neonatal foals. Management of this severe syndrome remains difficult, requiring intensive intervention. Key aspects of management include infection control, hemodynamic support, immunomodulatory interventions, and metabolic/endocrine support. Infection control largely consists of early antimicrobial therapy, plasma transfusions, and local therapy for the infected focus. In cases with severe sepsis or septic shock, hemodynamic support with fluids, vasoactive agents, and respiratory support insuring oxygen delivery to vital organs is important. Nutritional support is important, but close monitoring is needed to avoid hyperglycemia and hypoglycemia.

Some veterinarians describe particularly sick horses or neonatal foals as being endotoxemic, whereas others refer to the same animals as having the systemic inflammatory response syndrome. This article reviews the basis for the use of each of these terms in equine practice, and highlights the mechanisms underlying the response of the horse's innate immune system to key structural components of the microorganisms that initiate these conditions, including how some of those responses differ from other species. Current approaches used to treat horses with these conditions are summarized, and caution advised on extrapolating findings from other species to the horse.

hyperchloremia suggests that crystalloids with a lower chloride concentration may be more appropriate for use. Second, modifications to the understanding of the Starling equation suggest that the benefits of colloids may be more limited than previously thought. In addition, the negative effects of fluid overload on morbidity and mortality are becoming increasingly recognized. Although more specific research in horses is needed, these principles are likely to apply across all species.

Treatment of acute hemorrhage in the horse involves targeted medical management and also may involve surgical stabilization. This article provides an approach to the initial stabilization and information on available topical hemostats. The practice of blood collection and transfusion is also described, with attention to new information on viability of transfused equine blood, potential negative effects of blood transfusion, and methods of cell salvage.

Although primary coagulopathies are rare in horses, changes in coagulation and fibrinolysis are commonly associated with inflammatory diseases. A clear understanding of the pathophysiology of normal and abnormal hemostasis is required to be able to choose and interpret diagnostic tests evaluating coagulation and fibrinolysis. After diagnosis, treatment of the underlying disease must occur regardless of whether clinical manifestations (excessive bleeding or thrombosis) of the coagulopathy are present or not. Specific treatment may be initiated if there are clinical signs of coagulopathy.

Bullet wounds in horses can cause a wide array of injuries, determined by the type of projectile, the energy of the bullet on entry, and the type of tissue the bullet encounters. Treatment includes identification of all structures involved, debridement of the permanent cavity, and establishing adequate drainage. Bullet wounds should be treated as contaminated, and broad-spectrum antibiotics, including those with an anaerobic spectrum, are indicated. Although musculoskeletal injuries resulting from gunshots are most common in horses, they carry a good prognosis for survival and return to function.

There is a recognizable standard of practice for infection control in veterinary medicine. Effort must be given to control and prevention of infectious disease transmission within a facility and among animal populations. In the critical care setting, patients typically have a high degree of systemic illness and immune compromise, are commonly subjected to invasive procedures and placement of indwelling devices, and frequently receive antimicrobials and gastric protectants. Every equine critical care unit is distinctive in its physical and operational features and the types of patients that are managed. Infection control programs must therefore be tailored to each facility's needs.

VETERINARY CLINICS OF NORTH AMERICA: EQUINE PRACTICE

THE CLINICS ARE NOW AVAILABLE ONLINE!
Access your subscription at:
www.theclinics.com

Preface

Emergency and Critical Care

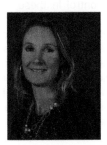
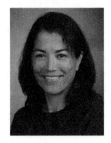

Vanessa L. Cook, VetMB, PhD, DACVS, DACVECC   Diana M. Hassel, DVM, PhD, DACVS, DACVECC

Editors

Ten years have passed since Dr Pamela Wilkins edited the last issue of *Veterinary Clinics of North America: Equine Practice* with the title, "Critical Care for All Ages." Much has changed since that 2004 issue, and the field of equine critical care has continued to grow. This has been reflected in the slow, but steady growth of large animal specialists within the American College of Veterinary Emergency and Critical Care. These *Veterinary Clinics of North America: Equine Practice* articles provide a unique perspective from textbook information as they represent the most up-to-date information from leaders in the field of equine critical care medicine and surgery. The goal of this issue is not to present a comprehensive overview of equine critical care and emergency topics, but rather to touch on highlights of critical care medicine that have not been recently reviewed, while not excluding some key, clinically relevant topics that may be immediately applied in the field. Unique topics that may not be found elsewhere, such as gunshot wounds in the horse as well as more advanced topics pertaining to physiology, systemic inflammatory response syndrome, and hemorrhage and blood transfusions, are also covered.

Among the more common conditions encountered by the emergency equine veterinarian are colic and neonatal triage. New information regarding pathogenesis, diagnostics, and therapy is available, so these and closely related topics are covered in depth. With the relatively recent RECOVER initiative pertaining primarily to small animal CPR, we felt it was appropriate to review the most recent and relevant techniques in equine CPR. This topic is further supported with a general review of triage in the neonatal foal as well as articles specific to management of neonatal sepsis and use and interpretation of blood lactate measurements in foals.

Our colic coverage includes a beautifully illustrated review of abdominal ultrasound; an article dedicated to the diagnostic workup and making the decision for referral; a review of the latest evidence-based information on crystalloid and colloid therapy; the use of lactate as a diagnostic tool; and diagnosis, pathogenesis, and treatment of coagulopathies.

Vet Clin Equine 30 (2014) xiii–xiv
http://dx.doi.org/10.1016/j.cveq.2014.06.001
0749-0739/14/$ – see front matter © 2014 Elsevier Inc. All rights reserved.

vetequine.theclinics.com

Coverage of the topic of critical care in the horse would not be complete without a review of infection control in equine critical care settings. Critically ill equine patients are particularly susceptible to health care–associated infections. The challenges of infection control as well as risks associated with management of critical care patients are covered along with guidelines to improve infection control in these high-risk settings.

We hope this issue on equine critical care provides an optimal combination of practical information and cutting-edge research to meet the needs of all veterinarians that are involved in the care of critically ill equine patients. A special thank-you is extended to the individual authors for their outstanding coverage of their respective topics. Each author is considered a leader in their respective field and we cannot thank them enough for their time and dedication to their contributions to this issue. We would also like to extend a sincere thank-you to Dr A. Simon Turner, for giving us the opportunity to collaborate on this edition dedicated to the equine critical care patient.

Vanessa L. Cook, VetMB, PhD, DACVS, DACVECC
Department of Large Animal Clinical Sciences
Michigan State University College of Veterinary Medicine
736 Wilson Road
East Lansing, MI 48824, USA

Diana M. Hassel, DVM, PhD, DACVS, DACVECC
Department of Clinical Sciences
College of Veterinary Medicine and Biological Sciences
Colorado State University
300 West Drake Road
Fort Collins, CO 80523-1678, USA

E-mail addresses:
vcook@cvm.msu.edu (V.L. Cook)
dhassel@colostate.edu (D.M. Hassel)

Field Triage of the Neonatal Foal

Elizabeth A. Carr, DVM, PhD

KEYWORDS

- Neonatal foal • Field triage • Sick • Recumbent • Weak

KEY POINTS

- When first evaluating a weak, recumbent, or lethargic foal on a farm it is often difficult to make a definitive diagnosis.
- The approach should be to treat what is treatable and prevent what is preventable.
- In many cases, the goal will be to stabilize a foal before referral to a tertiary care facility where more intensive and continuous treatment can be performed.

INTRODUCTION

The purpose of this article is to provide a quick reference for field triage of the sick neonatal foal. Therefore, information is focused toward diagnostics and treatments that can be performed in the field. When evaluating a weak, recumbent, or lethargic foal on the farm, it is often difficult to make a definitive diagnosis. Therefore, the approach should be to treat what is treatable and prevent what is preventable. In many cases, the goal will be to stabilize a foal before referral to a tertiary care facility where more intensive and continuous treatment can be performed.

PHYSICAL EXAMINATION OF THE NEWBORN FOAL

The normal foal should attempt to rise into sternal recumbency within seconds to minutes after delivery. On average, foals stand within 1 to 2 hours and nurse within 2 to 3 hours of birth. Mucous membranes and sclera may show the presence of ecchymotic hemorrhages caused by the pressure of passage through the birth canal and be mildly injected compared with adults. The capillary refill time is similar to adults. A normal cardiac sinus rhythm or sinus arrhythmia is ausculted. It is common to hear a systolic murmur (point of maximum intensity at the left heart base) for a few days after birth. Murmurs that persist longer should be evaluated further. The normal foal's respiratory rate and effort should decrease over the course of the first day of life,

The author has nothing to disclose.
Department of Large Animal Clinical Sciences, College of Veterinary Medicine, Michigan State University, 736 Wilson Road, East Lansing, MI 48824, USA
E-mail address: carreliz@cvm.msu.edu

and its heart rate should increase after a few minutes (**Table 1**). Foals should urinate within the first 24 hours of life, and urine should become progressively more dilute as they begin to consume a liquid diet. Newborn colts will occasionally be born with a persistent frenulum preventing them from dropping their penis to urinate. This condition is generally not a concern, as it will resolve over time. Many normal foals are born with a mild degree of carpal and fetlock valgus in their front limbs and slight varus in their hind fetlocks. This condition typically resolves as they grow. Foals should pass meconium, the first feces, within 12 to 24 hours. Meconium is dark brown to tan and may be hard or pasty. Subsequent milk feces are yellow tan and typically softer in consistency.

Neonates lack a menace response, as this is a learned behavior that will develop at a few weeks of life. Stimulation (auditory or visual) often results in exaggerated, jerky head movements. The neonatal foal's primary behavior should be directed toward maintaining close contact with its dam.

Foals should have a strong suckle reflex and nurse for relatively brief periods (minutes) as many as 8 times an hour. If a mare produces a large volume of milk, the foal may be unable to swallow it all and a small volume may be seen at its nostril after nursing. If persistent, this finding should trigger further evaluation to rule out dysphagia or a cleft palate.

Most lightweight foals will gain between 1 and 2 lb (0.5–1.0 kg) of weight per day. Foals that repeatedly return to the udder to nurse may be frustrated because of a lack of adequate milk production. Measurement of urine specific gravity and weight gain are important methods to determine adequate nutritional intake. Foals ingesting normal volumes of milk will have dilute urine (specific gravity 1.004–1.010). If a scale is not available, a string or weight tape can be used to measure change in body girth to assess daily weight gain.

Foals can be bradycardic at birth; the heart rate should increase relatively quickly to normal values. Persistent bradycardia can be caused by hypoxia, hypoglycemia, and hypothermia. Oxygen supplementation should be instituted. A continuous intravenous (IV) infusion of dextrose is recommended (see section on fluid therapy) if glucose monitoring is not available. Bolus therapy with glucose-containing fluids is not recommended, as hyperglycemia has deleterious effects. If bolus therapy is unavoidable, dextrose should be added to an isotonic crystalloid at a low percent (0.5% solution = 10 mL 50% glucose in 1-L crystalloids). If a foal is mildly hypothermic, it is recommended to allow slow, passive warming (cover the foal and keep in a dry, warm area out of the wind), as hypothermia is protective against hypoxic brain injury.[1] With more severe hypothermia, active warming is recommended and is best done by infusion of warmed IV fluids. The use of external heat sources is controversial as the resultant peripheral vasodilation can cause a reflex drop in core temperatures as cold blood flows centrally from the periphery.

The causes of tachycardia include pain, hypovolemia, anemia, fever, and excitement. If pain, fever, anemia, and excitement are ruled out, fluid therapy is indicated to attempt to correct hypovolemia (see section on IV fluid therapy).

Table 1
Physical examination findings in neonatal foals at birth, 2 to 4 hours, and 24 hours of age

Parameter	<10 min	2–4 h	24 h
Heart rate beats per min	40–60	100–200	80–120
Respiratory rate beats per min	40–60	20–40	20–40
Body temperature (F/C)	99–102/37–39	99–102/37–39	99–102/37–39

As the foal clears fluid from its lungs, its respiratory rate and effort should decline. Prominent rib retraction and the presence of an abdominal effort with paradoxic collapse of the chest wall during inspiration are indicators of respiratory distress and suggest respiratory or cardiac dysfunction. The foal's chest wall is extremely compliant compared with the adult animal. Respiratory muscle contraction is needed to maintain thoracic and lung volume and prevent alveolar collapse and atelectasis. Foals that are sick, weak, hypoglycemic, or have underlying respiratory disease may develop respiratory muscle exhaustion, worsening atelectasis, and pulmonary function.

During parturition, mucous membranes may appear gray or cyanotic; this should rapidly resolve once the foal is delivered. Pale mucous membranes can be an indicator of anemia or hypovolemic shock. Icteric mucous membranes can indicate hemolysis (neonatal isoerythrolysis), in utero placental dysfunction, or liver dysfunction. Further evaluation including blood work (complete blood count and serum chemistry analysis) and ultrasound examination looking for evidence of internal bleeding is recommended. Because cyanosis requires between 2 and 5 g of deoxygenated hemoglobin per deciliter of blood, anemic individuals may not be cyanotic even in the presence of severe hypoxia.[2] Petechia on the mucous membranes or ears can be an indicator of septicemia or thrombocytopenia.

Examination of the eye may aid the clinician in determining a diagnosis as hypopyon, or hyphema may be present in septic foals. Retinal hemorrhages may also be present in neonates born with equine herpesvirus type 1 infection. Sick foals may have abnormal blink responses or tear production making them more susceptible to corneal injury.

Dehydration and poor body fat stores can result in the development of entropion. If not recognized quickly, corneal abrasion and ulceration can develop. Treatment should be directed at correcting the abnormal lid position. This correction can be achieved by pulling the lid margin out to its normal position and placing a skin staple or mattress suture below and perpendicular to the lid margin to hold the lid out. Temporary correction can also be achieved by injecting 0.5 mL of procaine penicillin G subcutaneously approximately 5 mm below the lid margin. As the lid distends, the margin is rolled out and returned to its normal position. This technique may need to be repeated as the solution dissipates over time. Entropion usually resolves once the foal is rehydrated or gains weight.

Important Points
- The absence of cyanosis does not rule out hypoxia.
- The presence of hypopyon or hemorrhage in the eye is an indicator of sepsis.
- Persistent bradycardia or deterioration in respiratory rate or effort are signs of cardiopulmonary dysfunction and require immediate intervention.

Dysphagia/Loss of Suckle/Milk Regurgitation

The suckle reflex is one of the first things to deteriorate when a foal is sick. Clinical signs may include coughing after nursing, milk reflux at the nose, auscultation of milk in the trachea, and/or clinical signs of pneumonia. Causes of dysphagia or loss of the suckle include

- Perinatal asphyxia syndrome (PAS), Hypoxic ischemic encephalopathy (HIE)
- Sepsis
- Hypoglycemia
- Hypothermia

- Cleft palate
- Muscle dysfunction (selenium deficiency, glycogen branching enzyme deficiency)
- Hyperkalemic periodic paralysis

In some cases, the foal will appear to nurse normally but, lacking a competent suckle, will aspirate each time it drinks. When sick foals are fed via bottle or held up to nurse, they will often struggle and aspirate a portion of the meal. Auscultation of milk in the trachea during nursing is the most accurate way to assess dysphagia and milk aspiration.

The most common cause of dysphagia seems to be a temporary loss of neuromuscular coordination of the suckle reflex in sick or premature foals. In such cases, an endoscopic examination may reveal upper airway collapse and pharyngeal edema. A cleft palate can be identified by digital examination of the oral cavity unless the cleft is in the soft palate beyond the reach of the examiner. In such cases, endoscopy or a speculum examination may be needed to definitively diagnose the condition.

Regardless of the underlying cause, it is paramount to prevent nursing, as continued aspiration will result in pneumonia. If the foal is housed with its mare, it should be muzzled to prevent nursing and an indwelling nasogastric tube placed for feeding. Antimicrobial therapy is indicated if evidence of aspiration or sepsis is present. Most dysphagic foals resolve the dysfunction over time. The time to resolution varies from days to weeks; in rare cases, swallowing never normalizes. To minimize aspiration, foals with persistent dysphagia can be trained to drink out of a bucket placed on the ground.

TRIAGE OF THE WEAK NEONATAL FOAL

Facing a recumbent, weak, neonatal foal can be overwhelming. Teasing out the cause or causes without immediate access to diagnostic tools and laboratory assessment can be difficult. The most common causes of weakness and the inability to rise or nurse are sepsis, PAS, and prematurity/dysmaturity. The assessment and treatment should be directed at both the treatment of problems and the prevention of potential complications. If a foal fails to respond or if other factors impact the ability to treat the foal at the farm, referral is indicated. Treatment recommendations include both therapy for specific conditions and general treatment of the weak, recumbent neonate.

Sepsis

Sepsis is the leading cause of foal mortality. Sepsis may develop in utero or after foaling. Clinical signs will depend on the organ systems affected as well as the duration and severity. In the early hyperdynamic stage, foals may be lethargic, have a poor suckle reflex, and injected hyperemic mucous membranes. Petechial hemorrhages may be present on the membranes or pinnae. A decreased capillary refill time, tachycardia, and tachypnea may be present. A fever may or may not be present. As sepsis progresses, the foal becomes progressively more depressed or obtunded. Poor cardiac output results in cool extremities, tachycardia, prolonged capillary refill time, and poor peripheral pulses. Hypothermia and hypoglycemia may develop. The common clinicopathologic abnormalities seen with sepsis include leucopenia, neutropenia, and hypoglycemia. With profound hypoglycemia or respiratory compromise, hypoxemia, hypercapnia, and a mixed acidosis may be seen.

PAS

The underlying pathologic process in PAS is thought to be the result of prolonged or severe tissue hypoxia. Hypoxia may occur during pregnancy, parturition, or immediately after foaling. Decreased energy supply results in loss of membrane pumps, loss of ion gradients, calcium influx, activation of calcium-dependent enzymes and cellular damage.[3] Subsequent reperfusion can result in further damage via production of reactive oxygen species and inflammatory changes. Foals affected with PAS may be normal at birth and gradually become disinterested in their dams as cerebral swelling and cellular injury progresses. They may lose their suckle reflex and become excessively sleepy and difficult to rouse. Severe cases may become recumbent, progress to seizures, and develop an abnormal, apneustic pattern of breathing. Gastrointestinal signs may vary from mild feed intolerance to colic, gas distension, and bloody diarrhea. Many affected foals fail to urinate in response to bladder distension and require catheterization of the bladder to prevent rupture. Additional clinical signs will vary depending on organ system dysfunction.

Most foals affected with PAS will recover with supportive care and time. The goals of treatment of PAS are to prevent further cellular injury; control seizures and other effects of organ dysfunction; and prevent secondary problems, such as sepsis.

Prematurity/Dysmaturity

Prematurity is defined as a foal born with a gestational age of less than 320 days. Dysmaturity is defined as a foal born after a normal gestation length (320 days or more) that exhibits the physical characteristics of prematurity.

Clinical signs
- Small body stature, fine, silky hair coat, floppy ears, flaccid lips, domed forehead
- Tendon laxity and incomplete ossification of the cuboidal bones
- May see inverted neutrophil (N) to lymphocyte (L) ratio (normal N/L 2:1, affected foals ≤1:1)

Foals may be weak and unable to stand without assistance and have a poor suckle and poor tolerance to enteral feeding. Premature foals are often unable to regulate their body temperature or blood glucose. The premature intestinal tract may lack the specialized enterocytes necessary to absorb colostral antibodies, putting them at risk for failure of passive transfer (FPT) even after colostral ingestion.

Specific Treatment of Sepsis

- Broad-spectrum or culture-targeted antimicrobials
  - Gentamicin 12 mg/kg every 36 hours (first 2 weeks of life). Caution: nephrotoxicity
  - Amikacin 25 mg/kg every 24 hours (first 2 weeks of life). Caution: nephrotoxicity
  - Potassium+ penicillin 22,000 IU IV every 6 hours
  - Ceftiofur 2 to 10 mg/kg IV every 6 hours, intramuscular (IM) route every 12 hours
  - Trimethoprim-sulfonamide 30 mg/kg by mouth every 12 hours; avoid with gastrointestinal disease
  - Ticarcillin/clavulanic acid 50 to 100 mg/kg IV every 6 hours
- Antiinflammatory
  - Flunixin meglumine 0.25 to 1.1 mg/kg every 12 to 24 hours

Specific Treatment of PAS

- Further deterioration of the central nervous system (CNS) should be prevented, and seizures should be controlled.
- Secondary infection should be prevented with broad-spectrum antimicrobials.

- Perfusion and oxygen delivery should be maintained. Fluid therapy should be carefully calculated to maintain perfusion but not overhydrate, as overhydration can lead to cerebral edema and worsen neurologic dysfunction.
- Cerebral edema should be controlled. Mannitol (0.25–1.0 g/kg as a 20% solution over 20-minute infusion) will often result in neurologic improvement (temporary in individual cases).
- Respiratory compromise
  - Hypoxemia-bilateral nasal oxygen insufflations at 5 L/min
  - Hypoventilation or apneustic breathing pattern: caffeine loading dose 10 mg/kg by mouth followed by 2.5 to 3.0 mg/kg by mouth once a day to twice a day; if unsuccessful, may require mechanical ventilation

Specific Treatment of Prematurity

- Incomplete ossification of cuboidal bones: Lateral and anteroposterior radiographs of the carpus and tarsus should be performed to evaluate for incomplete ossification of the cuboidal bones. Weight bearing should be limited in affected cases to prevent the crush of the cartilaginous precursors. The crush of the tarsal and carpal bones can result in juvenile arthritis and have long-term catastrophic effects on the foal's athletic career; therefore, serial radiographs are important to monitor the ossification process.
- FPT should be assessed/treated.

GENERAL THERAPY FOR THE WEAK RECUMBENT FOAL

Broad-spectrum antimicrobial therapy is recommended in any weak recumbent foal to prevent or treat infection or sepsis.

Hypoglycemia is a frequent problem in the sick neonate. Many septic foals will have episodes of both hypoglycemia and hyperglycemia. If unable to tolerate oral feeding, institute IV nutritional support (see section on partial parenteral nutrition).

Nutrition Support

The healthy, full-term neonate is born with enough body fat and glycogen reserves to provide an energy supply for 12 to 24 hours. Premature or systemically compromised foals (eg, in utero sepsis) may lack these minimal reserves, making them at an increased risk for hypoglycemia, hypothermia, and organ dysfunction. The enteral route of nutrition is always preferred over parenteral, as enteral feeding has been shown to increase gastrointestinal mass and function compared with the parenteral route.[4] Unfortunately, the sick neonatal foal may be unable to tolerate enteral feeding. Enteral feeding should be avoided in severely hypotensive or hypothermic foals. Foals with enteropathy, whether secondary to oxygen deprivation or infection, may be unable to absorb nutrients and develop colic and diarrhea when fed. A detailed history and careful repeat assessments of the neonate's gastrointestinal tract (including ultrasound examination if possible) is critical to ensure that the foal is able to tolerate enteral feedings. The measurement of abdominal size can be useful to assess gastrointestinal distension. Colic signs in foals are often subtle; foals may appear fussy or agitated and show an increase in heart rate and respiratory rate. If deterioration is noted, enteral feeding should be discontinued or decreased until resolution.

Generally, a foal that is too sick to stand is also unlikely to have an adequate suckle reflex. Small, soft nasogastric tubes are available that may be sutured in place for longer-term use (MILA International Inc, Erlanger, KY). Before feeding, it is important to determine if the tube is in the stomach. If the foal is less than 24 hours of age, colostrum should be fed to provide both systemic and local passive immunity. It is generally best to start with small-volume feeding; if tolerated, the volume of feedings can be gradually increased every 1 to 2 feedings with an initial target goal of 10% body weight in milk per day. This volume equates to the approximate metabolic require-ments of a sick, recumbent foal maintained in a relatively warm, draft-free environ-ment.[5,6] Colic, bloating, increased gastric residuals, diarrhea, and ultrasound findings of ileus suggest intolerance to enteral feeding and should result in decreasing or temporarily discontinuing enteral feeding.

Assessment of the gastrointestinal tract before enteral feeding
- Borborygmi present
- Evidence of passage of gas or meconium
- Gastric residuals ≤60 mL
- Ultrasound findings of motility without evidence of intestinal distension

Partial parenteral nutrition
If enteral nutrition is not tolerated, an IV dextrose infusion should be instituted. The placenta supplies approximately 4 to 8 mg/kg/min of glucose, and this is a useful target when providing short-term parenteral support. This rate would equate to 4 to 8 mL of a 5% dextrose solution per minute. Glucose infusion alone is inadequate as a long-term nutritional source, and more complete parenteral nutrition is needed with prolonged intolerance to enteral feeding.

> For example, a 50-kg, 1-day-old foal presents recumbent and weak with signs of sepsis. The phys-ical examination reveals the presence of auscultable borborygmi. The ultrasound examination reveals a normal stomach size, normal-sized small intestine with decreased (but present motility), normal intestinal wall thickness, and no evidence of gas in the intestinal walls. A nasogastric tube is placed, and the aspiration to assess gastric residuals is negative. Approximately 60 mL of milk is given via the nasogastric (NG) tube. If the foal tolerates the feeding (no colic signs and <40 mL residual on subsequent NG tube aspiration), an additional 100 mL is fed 1 to 2 hours later. The goal is to reach approximately 400 mL every 2 hours (10% of body weight) over a 24-hour period. If unable to reach this goal within 24 hours, consider the addition of parenteral nutrition.

  With appropriate medical care, most sick neonates will begin to gain weight when provided 10% of its body weight in milk daily (**Table 2**). The healthy term foal ingests approximately 15% of its body weight in milk daily, this increases to 20% to 30% over the first few weeks of life. As a foal becomes stronger and more active, the amount fed should be gradually increased to normal volumes. The failure to gain weight can be a sign of uncontrolled illness, such as a focus of infection, or be the result of insufficient nutritional support.

Enteral feeds
Mare's milk or colostrum is ideal enteral feed. The mare's milk contains approximately 500 to 600 kcal/L, whereas colostrum contains approximately 1000 kcal/L. In contrast

Table 2 Milk intake volumes for a 50-kg foal		
Body Weight in Milk/d (%)	L/d	Feedings (mL/2 h)
5	2.5	208
10	5.0	420
15	7.5	630

to milk, mare's milk replacer is high in potassium and low in sodium and chloride. When using a milk replacer, it is important to provide a fresh-water source to avoid the risk of hypernatremia caused by the excess salt ingestion. A milk replacer designed for foals is ideal to ensure adequate protein, fat, and carbohydrates. Most of the ingredients should be milk based rather than plant based.

FPT

A complete failure is immunoglobulin G (IgG) less than 400.
A partial failure is IgG greater than 400 and less than 800.

Causes of FPT include
- A lack of colostral antibody in the first milk can be caused by loss (dripping) before foaling or inadequate production (primiparous and aged, debilitated mares at greater risk).
- Failure to ingest colostrum may be caused by the foal's inability to stand and nurse (caused by illness or musculoskeletal problems) during the critical 24-hour period.
- Failure to absorb colostrum may be caused by delayed ingestion (loss of specialized enterocytes) or because of prematurity/dysmaturity/in utero illness (lack of development of specialized enterocytes before birth).

Treatment
- At less than 24 hours of age, feed good-quality colostrum (good-quality colostrum [high in IgG] specific gravity $\geq$1.060 [using a colostrometer] or 23% refractive index [using a sugar refractometer]).
- At greater than 24 hours of age, perform a plasma transfusion. The rule of thumb is that approximately 1 L of plasma will increase the IgG to 200 mg/dL in a healthy foal and 100 mg/dL in a septic foal.
- If plasma is not an option, treat the foal with broad-spectrum antimicrobials.

IV Fluid Support of the Foal

Signs of poor perfusion and hypovolemia in the sick neonate may be caused by decreased fluid volume, inadequate cardiac function (poor contractility), or vascular changes (vasoactive shock), which can result from prolonged hypoxia, hypoglycemia, or sepsis. The placement of a jugular catheter and fluid boluses of 10 to 20 mL/kg of an isotonic crystalloid over a 20-minute period are recommended. Glucose-containing fluids should never be used as bolus fluids, as hyperglycemia (and potentially rebound hypoglycemia) will result. The reevaluation of the foal's cardiovascular status should be performed after each bolus. If no improvement is noted, a second (or third) bolus may be given until the maximum central venous pressure (CVP) is reached (8–10 cm of water). It is difficult to measure CVP in a field situation; consequently, a maximum of 3 fluid boluses is usually recommended to avoid fluid overload. Foals that fail to respond are likely to have cardiac or vascular dysfunction and require more intensive medical support including vasopressor therapy. Such cases are best referred to a neonatal intensive care facility.

Maintenance fluid therapy

The neonatal foal cannot be managed as a small version of the adult horse when calculating fluid therapy. The foal's kidneys are less effective in excreting sodium and water, and its vascular permeability is increased compared with the adult. Further, the septic foal or foal with ischemic injury may have abnormal responses to fluid fluxes, such as the syndrome of inappropriate antidiuretic hormone secretion resulting in further inability to handle excess fluid infusions. Overhydration can result in edema, vascular volume expansion, and excess weight gain. Edema affects oxygen delivery and can exacerbate existing organ dysfunction.

In human and many equine neonatal units, the approach to fluid therapy has shifted to one of fluid and sodium restriction. Fluid therapy is calculated based on body mass and surface area (**Table 3**). Sodium intake is restricted to approximately 3 mg/kg/d to attempt to avoid sodium excess. Continuous rate infusions of 5% dextrose with supplemental electrolytes are best used. Remember to include medications when calculating sodium intake.

For example, the following is a calculation for a 47-kg foal:

10 kg × 100 mL/kg/d = 1000 mL

10 kg × 50 mL/kg/d = 500 mL

27 kg × 25 mL/kg/d = 675 mL

= 2175 mL/d or ~90 mL/h

Using this fluid-restricted plan, urine specific gravity should not be diluted as seen with a healthy foal on a milk diet. If the foal is being supplemented with enteral feeding, the fluid calculations should be adjusted. It is important to adjust this rate if increased losses are present.

Supportive Care

Pressure sores may develop if not kept well bedded, cleaned, and repositioned frequently. Corneal ulcers can result from decreased tear production or trauma caused by accumulation of bedding/debris in the eye. Foals lying in lateral recumbency for prolonged periods will develop atelectasis of the dependant lung. Atelectasis will exacerbate the existing lung disease and affect oxygen delivery. The Pao_2 can decrease by as much as 15 mm Hg when switching a foal from sternal to lateral recumbency; therefore, it is important to try to keep foals in sternal recumbency to maintain lung volume, for ventilation/perfusion matching, and to maximize oxygen delivery to the tissues.

Respiratory Support

Physical examination findings of respiratory distress indicate the need for further assessment of pulmonary function. Oxygen insufflations should be instituted until further monitoring can be performed. A soft, rubber Foley catheter can be slid up the ventral meatus (to the level of the medial canthus) to facilitate oxygen supplementation; 5 L/min of oxygen insufflations is recommended. In foals exhibiting severe hypoxemia, bilateral insufflations may be necessary (5 L in each nostril). Humidification is

Table 3	
Maintenance fluid therapy for the neonatal foal	
First 10 kg body weight	100 mL/kg/d
Second 10 kg body weight	50 mL/kg/d
Additional kg body weight	25 mL/kg/d

recommended for long-term oxygen insufflations but is not necessary in the short-term while stabilizing a foal for transport.

Important points
- Weak, recumbent foals are at risk for hypoglycemia, which may exacerbate the underlying problems.
- Supportive care is critical to the long-term recovery.
- Do not enterally feed a hypothermic hypotensive foal. Carefully monitor the gastrointestinal response when starting enteral nutrition in the critically ill neonatal foal.

OTHER COMMON DISORDERS OF THE NEONATE
Neonatal Isoerythrolysis

Clinical signs of neonatal isoerythrolysis may include lethargy, tachycardia, tachypnea, pale mucous membranes with/without icterus. The onset of clinical signs varies from 1 to 7 days of age and depends on the rapidity and severity of hemolysis. Mule foals are overrepresented.

Treatment
- Blood transfusion is recommended in severely anemic foals or for those foals that are so weak that they are unwilling to nurse. The goal of transfusion is to provide oxygen-carrying capacity until a regenerative response occurs. Crossmatching is ideal; if it is unavailable, transfusion from an Aa Qa blood type negative gelding is recommended.
- Dexamethasone 0.08 mg/kg IV or IM in peracute cases may decrease hemolysis.
- Supportive care includes the following:
  ○ Nasogastric intubation and feeding if foal is too weak to nurse
  ○ Broad-spectrum antimicrobials

Disorders of the Lungs

Pneumonia
The most common cause of respiratory compromise/distress is bacterial pneumonia. This condition may result from aspiration or bacteremia. Radiographs reveal the presence of consolidation, most commonly in the cranioventral lung fields, though a diffuse pattern may be seen with hematogenous pneumonia. Thoracic ultrasound examination typically reveals the presence of pleural irregularities and consolidating lesions. Pleural effusion is rare with neonatal pneumonia. Foals with viral pneumonia usually present with severe dyspnea and high fevers and have a very characteristic ultrasound pattern consisting of wide-spread, diffuse pleural irregularities or comet tails and small consolidated (fluid density) lesions.

A tracheal wash with bacterial culture and sensitivity is recommended to ensure appropriate antimicrobial therapy. However, a transtracheal wash should not be performed in foals with signs of respiratory distress, as it may lead to further deterioration and collapse.

Treatment Broad-spectrum antimicrobial therapy is indicated unless culture and sensitivity is available (see "Specific Treatment of Sepsis"). Foals should be maintained in sternal recumbency to maximize oxygenation and delivery. Foals that are in respiratory distress may be unwilling to nurse; in such cases, placement of an indwelling nasogastric tube is recommended to ensure nutritional support. Nasal oxygen supplementation is recommended if Pa_{O_2} decreases to less than 65 mm Hg (approximately equal to an arterial oxygen saturation less than 90%). Bilateral nasal insufflations at 5 L/min can increase inspired oxygen content as high as 49%.[7] A humidifier should be attached for long-term oxygen insufflations. Ventilatory support is recommended if $Paco_2$ is 65 mm Hg or greater. Caffeine is not recommended, as ventilatory failure is usually caused by respiratory muscle failure not neurologic dysfunction. Coupage of the thorax multiple times a day may help to break up and clear the debris within the lung. Keeping the foal well hydrated will also help in the clearance of inspissated material.

Apneustic breathing

The most common cause of apneustic or an irregular breathing pattern is perinatal asphyxia syndrome. Lack of oxygen delivery results in damage and depression of the respiratory center in the medulla. Other potential causes include hypoglycemia, hypothermia, and other forms of CNS disease (eg, meningitis, trauma). Botulism may also result in a weak, abnormal breathing pattern and hypercapnia but is frequently associated with muscle fasciculations and other signs of muscle weakness.

Treatment

- Treat the underlying disorder (hypoglycemia, hypothermia).
- For caffeine, the recommended loading dose is 10 mg/kg by mouth followed by 2.5 to 3.0 mg/kg once daily. The loading dose may result in significant stimulation in the neonate. An increase in the respiratory rate and effort indicates pulmonary or cardiac dysfunction.
- If hypoventilation persists, ventilatory support is recommended.

Disorders of the Umbilicus and Urinary Tract

The umbilical stalk will typically detach once the foal or mare stands. If bleeding occurs, a temporary clamp or umbilical tape may be applied. A 1:4 chlorhexidine solution or a 2% iodine solution is recommended as the umbilical dips. Stronger iodine solutions should be avoided, as they can scald the skin, cause edema, and cause early separation of the external umbilical stalk, which may predispose to the development of a patent urachus.

Patent urachus

Patent urachus may be present at birth or develop in foals that are recumbent for prolonged periods.

Treatment

- Broad-spectrum antimicrobials
- Phenazopyridine if excessive straining or cystitis/urachitis
- If severe or associated with infection, surgical removal may be indicated

Omphalophlebitis

Infections of the structures of the umbilical cord are relatively common in sick neonates and can result in secondary dissemination to other organ systems, including the lungs, joints, and bones. An ultrasound examination of the umbilical structures evaluating the size and echogenicity should be performed in any sick neonate.

Treatment

- Surgical removal
- Medical management with broad-spectrum or culture-directed antimicrobials

Dysuria

Foals that are weak and recumbent may not have the normal neurologic trigger to urinate when their bladder is distended. It is important to monitor urination and/or bladder size (via ultrasound exam) in all sick, recumbent foals to prevent this complication. In suspect cases a urinary catheter and closed collection system can be placed to prevent distension and rupture.

Urinary tract rupture and uroabdomen

Urinary bladder rupture can occur in utero, during foaling, or after birth in the neurologically impaired neonate. Clinical signs become apparent as urine accumulates, azotemia develops, and electrolyte derangements occur.

Clinical signs Clinical signs will depend on the location of the rupture, its duration, and the volume of urine accumulated. If the rupture of a ureter occurs, urine may accumulate in the retroperitoneal space but not in the peritoneal space.

Common findings include
- Pendulous, fluid-filled abdomen
- Tachycardia, tachypnea, lethargy, and weakness
- Decreased appetite and decreased suckle
- Respiratory compromise worsens as intra-abdominal pressure increases
- Pleural effusion may develop; urine may accumulate in the scrotum or ventral abdomen
- Straining to urinate
- With/without signs of sepsis

Diagnosis
- Ultrasound examination shows evidence of fluid within the peritoneal space.
- Peritoneal fluid creatinine is 2-fold or greater of blood creatinine.
- Serum chemistry analysis shows azotemia (creatinine usually elevated to a greater degree than blood urea nitrogen) hyperkalemia, +/− hyponatremia, hypochloremia, hypoxemia, and acidosis. (Electrolyte values will vary depending on the severity and duration of rupture and whether the foal has received prior fluid therapy support.)[8]

Treatment The initial treatment is aimed at stabilizing patients before referral for surgical correction. Although resolution with medical therapy has been reported, most cases require surgical repair of the tear. Hyperkalemia can be life threatening when it is 5.5 mEq/L or greater and must be addressed before surgical correction; this can best be achieved by the following:

- Drainage of the uroabdomen can be performed using a 14F or 16F Foley catheter, IV catheter, or chest tube. The catheter can be sutured in place to allow continued or repetitive drainage; however, it is important to know that they often become obstructed by fibrin or omentum necessitating their removal.
- Perform IV crystalloid therapy to normalize electrolyte derangements. The replacement volume should be at least equal to or exceed the volume of urine drained to prevent acute hypotension as abdominal pressure decreases.
- Sodium bicarbonate may be added to the saline infusion to lower serum potassium levels, as it results in intracellular movement of potassium. Calcium gluconate added to saline (separately from bicarbonate) will reduce the impact of hyperkalemia on cardiac function. An insulin and dextrose infusion will also help lower potassium levels, as glucose uptake is coupled to potassium uptake.
- Pleural effusion will generally resolve after abdominal drainage, though it may take several hours to days. Because pleural effusion can cause pulmonary atelectasis and affect respiratory function, it is recommended to delay anesthesia and surgical repair until the effusion has resolved.
- Broad-spectrum antimicrobial therapy is recommended postoperatively.

Disorders of the Musculoskeletal System

Flexor tendon laxity

Mild flexor tendon laxity will usually resolve with time and controlled exercise. Foals that are walking on their fetlocks or unable to stand because of severe laxity may require the placement of shoes with heel extensions and controlled, limited exercise until the laxity resolves. A light wrap may be applied to the fetlock to prevent abrasions. However, thicker support wraps should be avoided, as these will exacerbate the tendon laxity.

Flexural deformities (contracted tendons): Flexural deformities are thought to arise because of uterine malposition, ingestion of toxic plants, nutritional deficiencies, infections, and genetic defects.

Treatment

- The goal of therapy is to achieve tendon loading and stretch.
- Mild: The treatment includes physical therapy, support wraps, or splints and controlled exercise.
- Moderate: The treatment includes bandages and splints, with a daily bandage change and physical therapy.
- Severe: Surgical release may be necessary in severe cases
- The stretching of these tendons is painful, and analgesia and gastric ulcer prophylaxis is recommended.
- Oxytetracycline (2 to 3 g IV once) has been shown to result in a temporary increase in joint extension.

Avoid oxytetracycline in sick, dehydrated, hypovolemic foals or in those with signs of renal compromise.

Limit exercise, as foals can get tired and stumble increasing the risk of injury to the extensor tendons.

Septic arthritis/septic osteomyelitis

Clinical signs The earliest sign of septic arthritis or osteomyelitis is often lameness. Warmth, swelling, and pain may be palpated over the affected area, though these signs may be less obvious with osteomyelitis. Complete blood counts typically reveal an elevated white blood cell count (WBC) and fibrinogen. Foals may or may not have a fever. Regular palpation and assessment of gait is important, as early detection and treatment are factors in the prognosis for athleticism.

Diagnosis septic arthritis/osteomyelitis

- Synovial fluid cytology: A WBC greater than 30,000/µl, greater than 90% neutrophils, and total solids greater than 2.5 g/dL are consistent with sepsis. The absence of bacteria does not rule out the septic process.
- The presence of hyperfibrinogenemia and leukocytosis.
- Synovial fluid culture: *A negative culture does not rule out septic process.
- Radiographs of the affected region are recommended to evaluate for septic physitis or osteomyelitis. *Radiographs of the unaffected limb should be taken for comparison, as the normal foal's physes can appear irregular.

Treatment septic arthritis

- Lavage the affected joint with 1 to 2 L of an isotonic crystalloid solution (pH ~ 7.0). Every other day, lavage is recommended until cytology and clinical signs improve. In cases with excess fibrin and purulent debris, arthroscopy or arthrotomy may be necessary to more effectively debride the joint.

- Broad-spectrum antimicrobial therapy: Treatment for 3 to 6 weeks may be necessary. If an arthrotomy is performed, antimicrobial therapy should be maintained until the joint seals.
- Nonsteroidal antiinflammatory therapy: Treatment is recommended until inflammatory process has improved.
- Prophylactic antiulcer therapy is recommended in foals with painful conditions and those receiving nonsteroidal antiinflammatory therapy.

Treatment septic osteomyelitis
- Medical therapy is similar to that for septic arthritis.
- Aspiration and culture of the infected bone is recommended for more directed therapy.
- Regional limb perfusion with an aminoglycoside is useful to achieve high concentrations of antimicrobials at the site of infection. Use approximately one-third of the total daily dose, and decrease the daily IV dose accordingly to prevent overdosing.
- Surgical debridement may be performed.

Rib fractures
Rib fractures can occur without any history of dystocia or trauma. The signs of rib fractures may include tachypnea (often shallow rapid breathing), tachycardia, chest wall edema +/− crepitus at the fracture site, and clinical signs of hemorrhage. Auscultation over the fracture site may reveal a click that occurs with the respiratory cycle. Most rib fractures occur near the costochondral junction and are best visualized by ultrasound examination using a linear probe placed parallel with and on top of the rib.

Treatment
- Limited exercise/stall rest for 3 to 4 weeks
- Surgical stabilization if unstable or displaced fragments

DISORDERS OF THE GASTROINTESTINAL TRACT
Colic

Colic signs in a foal can be subtle; foals may appear agitated, unable to settle, and have an increased heart and respiratory rate. They may flag their tail and stomp a foot. With severe pain, signs become more obvious. The evaluation of the colicky foal should include a physical examination, careful history, digital rectal examination, passage of a nasogastric tube, and an abdominal ultrasound. The presence of gastric reflux suggests a small intestinal disorder.

Common causes of neonatal colic
Meconium impaction
Atresia coli
Ileocecocolic aganglionosis
Enterocolitis
Gastric ulcers
Bowel obstruction: intussusceptions, volvulus, strangulation, incarceration
Peritonitis: usually secondary to ruptured gastric ulcers, umbilical abscessation, or uroabdomen

Diagnostic aids for colic

- Nasogastric intubation should be performed to check for reflux and gastric distension secondary to outflow obstruction.
- Abdominal radiographs with or without contrast agents can be helpful to assess the location and type of distension and to evaluate for impaction or atresia.
- Abdominocentesis and cytologic evaluation should be performed to diagnose peritonitis, ruptured bladder, or bowel.

Meconium impaction

Meconium impaction is the most common cause of colic in the neonatal foal. The clinical signs include decreased nursing, straining to defecate with an arched back, flagging of the tail, and a lack of meconium production. A digital examination may reveal hard fecal balls in the rectum. With complete obstruction, abdominal distension may develop. Severe distension can result in respiratory compromise. Radiographs or ultrasound may reveal fecal material in the distal colon or rectum. A barium enema can be performed for further evaluation and to attempt to rule out focal atresia of the intestinal tract.

Treatment A warm water enema (using ~150 mL of warm water) can be performed in the standing foal using gentle restraint. A polyurethane stallion urinary catheter or an enema tube can be used. The tip of the tube should be lubricated and gently inserted until resistance is felt. Water can be infused by gravity while gently manipulating the tube to try to advance around the impaction. The addition of a small amount of dish soap may help resolve the impaction; however, repeated infusion of soap can cause further irritation of the mucosa and may ultimately worsen the foal's discomfort.

An acetylcysteine retention enema is recommended for meconium impactions that do not resolve with a warm water enema. Sedation is recommended (diazepam 0.1 mg/kg IV) to keep the foal quite while the enema is infused. Once the foal is recumbent, a 30-cm^3 balloon 30F lubricated Foley catheter is placed, and the balloon is distended with saline. Elevating the foal's hind end will aid the gravity flow. After infusion, the catheter is clamped to retain the enema for a minimum of 15 minutes (ideal time is 30–45 minutes).

N-acetyl-ʟ-cysteine retention enema
If using Mucomyst (20% acetylcysteine): Add 40 mL of solution to 160 mL of warm water
If using powdered N-acetyl-ʟ-cysteine (NALC): Add 8 g of powdered NALC and 1.5 tbsp of baking soda to 200 mL of water.

Oral laxatives The use of oral laxatives, such as mineral oil, can be helpful, particularly with proximal impactions. Mineral oil (~60 mL) can be given by nasogastric tube. Mineral oil should never be given by syringe feeding, as aspiration will result. Detergents, such as dioctyl sodium sulfosuccinate (DSS), or castor oil are not recommended because they cause irritation to the intestinal mucosa and can result in further colic and diarrhea.

IV fluids With protracted impactions, IV fluids may be necessary to maintain hydration and aid in treatment.

Analgesics/prokinetics

- Nonsteroidal antiinflammatory drugs are potent analgesics. If they are used, it is critical to ensure adequate hydration to prevent renal toxicity and to institute gastroprotectant therapy to attempt to minimize the side effects.

- IM butorphanol (0.1 mg/kg) may provide analgesia. Combining it with diazepam (5–10 mg/50 kg foal) may provide sedation, allowing time for a retention enema or other treatment to take effect.
- Neostigmine (0.005–0.01 mg/kg IM or subcutaneous) has been effective in resolving meconium impactions and allowing passage of gas.

Atresia coli
Atresia can be a difficult disorder to definitively diagnose. The passage of meconium does not rule out an atresia coli. A barium enema followed by serial radiographic images may identify an area that is constricted or atretic. A definitive diagnosis may require surgical exploration. Reports of successful resection and anastomosis of atresia coli exist.[9]

Ileocecocolic aganglionosis (overo lethal white syndrome)
Ileocecocolic aganglionosis, or lethal white syndrome, is a genetic defect recognized in homozygous, overo, paint foals. Affected foals are usually completely white or have only small spots of color on their bodies. An endothelin receptor B mutation results in complete aganglionosis of the myenteric and submucosal ganglia of the intestinal tract.[10] Foals appear normal at birth but develop signs of colic, profound ileus, and intestinal distension. The diagnosis is made based on clinical signs coupled with ultrasonographic evidence of profound ileus and distension in white, homozygous, overo, paint foals. There is no treatment of this disorder, and euthanasia is recommended. A genetic test is available to identify heterozygous individuals.

Enterocolitis/diarrhea
The causes of enterocolitis and diarrhea include bacterial, viral, protozoal, nutritional, and ischemic (necrotizing enterocolitis) (**Table 4**). Bacterial causes include *Clostridium perfringens* type A and C, *Clostridium difficile*, salmonellosis, and, less commonly, *Escherichia coli*, *Bacteroides fragilis*, and *Aeromonas hydrophila*. Rotavirus is the most common viral cause, though coronavirus, adenovirus, and parvovirus have been isolated from foals. *Cryptosporidium* species have been isolated from foals with diarrhea but can also be isolated from normal foals. Nutritional causes include overfeeding, lactose intolerance, and sudden diet changes.

Because blood flow is shunted to vital organs during hypoxic/ischemic periods, foals with PAS or septic shock often have ischemic damage to their gastrointestinal tract. Clinical signs of ischemic enteropathy can range from mild colic and intolerance of enteral feeding to profound ileus, sepsis, and bloody diarrhea. Affected foals may present with other organ dysfunction. Sepsis may develop secondarily to bacterial translocation across the damaged gastrointestinal mucosal barrier.

Table 4
Fecal characteristics and diagnostic assays for common diarrheal causes in foals

Cause	Characteristics	Diagnosis
Clostridium perfringens	May be bloody or foul smelling	Culture and toxin assay
Clostridium difficile	May be bloody and foul smelling	Culture and toxin assay
Salmonella spp	May be bloody or foul smelling	Fecal culture
Rotavirus	Watery	ELISA assay for viral antigens
Lactose intolerance	Watery	Response to lactase supplementation
Overfeeding	Watery	Response to change in feeding regimen
Foal heat diarrhea	Transient, no other signs of illness	Timing with mare's heat cycle

When presented with a foal with enterocolitis and diarrhea, it is important to institute symptomatic treatment regardless of the cause. Foals with enterocolitis often do not tolerate oral feeding. Injured enterocytes may be unable to digest nutrients resulting in bacterial overgrowth in the large bowel, gas production, and further colic. Auscultation and ultrasound examination should be performed to assess motility. A nasogastric tube should be placed to check for reflux and gastric distension. Decreasing or temporarily stopping enteral feeding may be necessary, as feeding may exacerbate clinical signs. Symptomatic therapy includes

- IV fluid support (see section on IV fluid therapy)
- Withhold feeding until motility returns; gradual reintroduction to enteral feeding (see nutrition section)
- Broad-spectrum antimicrobial therapy: for diarrhea, consider addition of metronidazole 15 to 25 mg/kg every 6 hours
- Parenteral nutritional support (see section on nutritional support)
- Antiinflammatory therapy
- Gastric ulcer prophylaxis
- Lactase supplementation when reinstituting feeding

Nutritional causes of colic and diarrhea
Overfeeding Foals that quickly ingest large volumes of milk or milk replacer can develop gastric distension, colic, and diarrhea. Foals fed large volumes infrequently will consume the large volume rapidly; incomplete digestion results in bacterial overgrowth in the large intestine, resulting in colic, gas production, and diarrhea. Treatment is to decrease the volume ingested at each feeding. Feeding milk cold may help, as it is less palatable and may slow the foal down.

Lactose intolerance The most common cause of lactose intolerance is injury to and loss of enzyme-producing enterocytes. Supplementation with the enzyme lactase in each feeding is helpful in resolving clinical signs. Over time, as the intestinal tract heals, this syndrome typically resolves.

SEIZURES
Causes of Seizures

- Perinatal asphyxia syndrome
- Meningitis
- Trauma
- Idiopathic epilepsy of Arabian foals
- Congenital abnormalities: juvenile epilepsy, lavender foal syndrome, and glycogen branching enzyme deficiency

Clinical Signs

Seizures can be difficult to detect, as clinical signs may be subtle, including repetitive tremors, abnormal eye movements, hyperesthesia, excessive stretching, or extensor muscle tone when recumbent. Because secondary injury from excess neurotransmitter and calcium release can occur, it is critical to control seizures.

Treatment Options

- Diazepam: Administer diazepam 0.1 to 0.44 mg/kg IV bolus to effect (5–20 mg per 50-kg foal). Diazepam has a relatively short half-life, and the effect may be short lived, requiring additional therapy. Monitor for respiratory depression.

- Midazolam: Administer midazolam 0.04 to 0.1 mg/kg IV slowly (2–5 mg per 50-kg foal). Midazolam may be used as a continuous-rate infusion for long-term control at 2 to 5 mg/h. Monitor for respiratory depression.
- Phenobarbital: For persistent seizures uncontrolled by diazepam or midazolam, use phenobarbital 2 to 3 mg/kg IV.
- Propofol: Use propofol in cases that are refractory to the aforementioned medications at 4 mg/kg IV continuous-rate infusion.

For long-term control with refractory seizures

- Potassium bromide: Administer 60 to 90 mg/kg orally once daily.
- Magnesium infusion: Administer a loading dose of 50 mg/kg IV over 1 hour and a maintenance dosage of 25 mg/kg/h.

Additional Support for Seizures

If cerebral edema is present

- Administer mannitol 0.5 to 1.0 g/kg of 20% solution IV over 15 minutes; the dose may be repeated.
- Bandage the legs and pad the head to prevent injury. If the head protector is not available, wrap a protective bandage over the eyes (after placing lubricant) to avoid eye abrasions and corneal ulceration.
- Keep the head elevated to prevent increased intracranial pressure and exacerbation of cerebral edema.
- Avoid overhydration.

REFERENCES

1. Drury PP, Gunn ER, Bennet L, et al. Mechanisms of hypothermic neuroprotection. Brain Res 2014. http://dx.doi.org/10.1016/j.brainres.2014.03.023. pii:S0006-8993(14)00371-0.
2. Goss GA, Hayes JA, Burdon JG. Deoxyhaemoglobin concentrations in the detection of central cyanosis. Thorax 1988;43(3):212–3.
3. Wasnick G, Gunn ER, Drury PP, et al. The mechanisms and treatment of asphyxia encephalopathy. Front Neurosci 2014;8:40.
4. Burrin DG, Stoll B, Ruhong J, et al. Minimal enteral nutrient requirements for intestinal growth in neonatal piglets: how much is enough. Am J Clin Nutr 2000;71:1603–10.
5. Jose-Cunilleras E, Viu J, Corradini I, et al. Energy expenditure of critically ill neonatal foals. Equine Vet J Suppl 2012;(41):48–51.
6. Paradis MR. Caloric needs of the sick foal determined by the use of indirect calorimetry. Proc 3rd Dorothy Havemeyer Foundation Neonatal Septicemia Workshop. 2001:13–6.
7. Wong DM, Alcott CJ, Want C, et al. Physiologic effects of nasopharyngeal administration of supplemental oxygen at various flow rates in healthy neonatal foals. Am J Vet Res 2010;71:1081–8.
8. Kablack KA, Embertson RM, Bernard WV, et al. Uroperitoneum in the hospitalized equine neonate: retrospective study of 31 cases, 1988-1997. Equine Vet J 2000; 32:505–8.
9. Schneider JE, Leipold HW, White SL. Repair of congenital atresia of the colon in a foal. J Eq Sci 1981;1:121.
10. Santschi EM, Purdy AK, Valberg SJ, et al. Endothelin receptor B polymorphism associated with lethal white foal syndrome in horses. Mamm Genome 1998;9: 306–9.

CPR in the Neonatal Foal

Has RECOVER Changed Our Approach?

Jonna Maaria Jokisalo, DVM[a], Kevin Thomas Trent Corley, BVM&S, PhD, MRCVS[b],*

KEYWORDS

- Resuscitation • Cardiopulmonary arrest • Foal • Life support • Monitoring

KEY POINTS

- Respiratory arrest usually precedes cardiac arrest in the newborn foal.
- Team training and preparation is critical before resuscitation.
- Ventilation should be performed with short, infrequent breaths at a rate of 10 to 20 breaths per minute.
- In accordance with recommendations from RECOVER, a "push hard, push fast" approach should be used for chest compressions.
- If it proves necessary to use drugs during foal resuscitation, epinephrine is the principal drug used. A dose of 0.01 mg/Kg IV or 0.1 mg/Kg intratracheally should be used.

WHAT IS RECOVER?

RECOVER, The Reassessment Campaign on Veterinary Resuscitation, was created to optimize survival of small animal patients from cardiopulmonary arrest (CPA), and its aim was to improve preparedness and prevention measures, basic life support (BLS), advanced life support (ALS), and post-cardiac arrest (PCA) care. Before RECOVER, consensus-based guidelines for such strategies did not exist in veterinary medicine. The goal of RECOVER was therefore to systematically evaluate the evidence on clinical practice of veterinary cardiopulmonary resuscitation (CPR). The campaign was set up to devise clinical guidelines on how to best treat CPA in dogs and cats and also to identify important knowledge gaps in veterinary CPR that need to be filled to improve the quality of recommendations, and thus the quality of patient care in the future.[1]

Reported survival rates to hospital discharge after CPA occurring in the hospital differ greatly between small animal and humans. Less than 6% of dogs and cats have reported to survive to hospital discharge,[2–5] whereas the survival rate is approximately 20% in humans in a similar setting.[6,7] Studies looking at the survival rate to hospital discharge in horses experiencing CPA in hospital setting are lacking.

The authors have nothing to disclose.
[a] Animagi Hevossairaala Hyvinkää, Hyyppäräntie 41, Hyvinkää 05800, Finland; [b] Veterinary Advances Ltd, 9 Ballysax Hills, The Curragh, Co Kildare, Ireland
* Corresponding author.
E-mail address: kcorley@equineadvances.com

Frauenfelder[8] reported 75% success rate on external cardiovascular resuscitation in adult anesthetized ponies. Eight anesthetized ponies sustained unexpected cardiac arrest while being used in an endotoxin shock study. In 6 of these ponies, return of spontaneous circulation was achieved with the combination of external cardiac massage and ventilatory support. No longer-term data were published. Palmer[9] presented a case series of 83 hospitalized large animal neonates (80% foals) requiring ALS (assisted ventilation and cardiac support [cardiac compressions and/or drugs]). Depending on the underlying cause, the rate of return of spontaneous circulation (ROSC) was 40% to 90%.

CAUSES FOR CPA IN EQUINE NEONATES

Although there are many reasons for CPA in foals, respiratory arrest almost always precedes cardiac arrest in the newborn foal. Premature placental separation, early severance or twisting of the umbilical cord, prolonged dystocia, or airway obstruction by fetal membranes are the most common reasons causing asphyxia in a neonatal foal, which can result in respiratory arrest. However, some foals do not start spontaneously breathing without any apparent birthing problem. Other causes for CPA in neonatal foals, not associated with birth, include primary lung disease leading to hypoventilation and hypoxia, septic shock, hypovolemia, metabolic acidosis, hyperkalemia, vasovagal reflex, hypoglycemia, and hypothermia. CPA resulting from tension pneumothorax and trauma has also been reported in foals.[10] Unlike in adult humans, cardiac arrest in neonatal foals is usually secondary to other systemic conditions, such as septic shock or respiratory failure, and not caused by primary cardiac failure; this explains why ventricular fibrillation (VF) is not a common presenting arrhythmia. In the rare occasions where CPA is cardiac in origin, it is usually secondary to hypoxic-ischemic or cytokine-mediated myocardial damage, congenital cardiac defects, myocarditis, endocarditis with coronary artery embolism, or cardiac tamponade.

CPR TRAINING AND TEAM DYNAMICS

It is important to recognize early which foals require resuscitation. If resuscitation is begun before a nonperfusing cardiac rhythm develops, the likelihood of revival is good (survival rate as high as 50%). If resuscitation efforts are delayed until after development of asystole, however, a less than 10% survival rate is to be expected.[10] Clinical human studies have shown that training people to recognize the signs of cardiac arrest improves the ability of first responders to recognize the need for CPA.[11] Cardiopulmonary resuscitation (CPR) given to patients not in CPA has been reported not to result in major harm.[12] Therefore, veterinary hospitals should teach all employees CPR and repeat training before every breeding season.

It is especially important to recognize the foals needing resuscitation at birth, because the foal may have arrested during the birthing process and therefore have had a prolonged period of arrest. For this reason, it is important to be familiar with the normal events at birth. The average length of Stage II of labor is 16.7 minutes.[13,14] The normal foal takes a few gasps initially but should be breathing regularly within 30 seconds of birth. The heart rate averages 70 bpm immediately after birth. Normal foals may have cardiac arrhythmias during the first hour of life.[15] Foals should have pain and sensory awareness at birth, develop a righting reflex with 5 minutes and a suck reflex within 2 to 20 minutes.

Severe respiratory distress, large abdominal effort, and open mouth breathing can occur immediately after birth from several congenital upper respiratory conditions, including bilateral choanal atresia, stenotic nares, and dorsal displacement of the soft palate, necessitating immediate placement of an endotracheal tube *per os* or emergency tracheostomy. An important differential for dyspnea immediately after birth is perinatal equine herpesvirus 1 infection. Persistently abnormal heart rates and arrhythmias require further investigation with an electrocardiogram (ECG).

Newborn foals require resuscitation if
- Gasping for longer than 30 seconds
- Respiratory movements or heart beat are absent
- The heart rate is less than 50 bpm and falling
- There is obvious dyspnea

Hospitalized foals require resuscitation if
- The heart rate is less than 50 bpm and falling
- There is apnea

Decreases in venous oxygen saturation, end-tidal carbon dioxide ($EtCO_2$) concentration, and muscle tone may be early signs of arrest.

Preparation

The most important step in resuscitation is thorough preparation. At the critical moment, there is no time to start looking for equipment or to try to remember CPR algorithms let alone drug doses. Everything that is needed for resuscitation should be easily accessible and able to be moved quickly to the stall side. The best way to achieve this is to organize a crash cart to be always kept in the same place in the hospital or car so it is easily found when needed. This crash cart should be checked before each breeding season and after every use so that it is ready when needed.

CPR—BASIC AND ADVANCED LIFE SUPPORT

CPR can be divided in three phases: BLS, ALS, and monitoring. Veterinary BLS consists of intubation, ventilation, and chest compressions. These include the recognition of CPA—or in foals, recognition of respiratory arrest—airway management, provision of ventilation, and chest compressions. BLS is the immediate response to CPA, and in humans and in some aspects also small animals, lay rescuers and medical professionals alike may accomplish most aspects. Numerous human and animal experimental studies have shown that the quality of BLS performed is associated with ROSC and survival in arrest victims.[16] BLS differs from the 2 other parts of CPR as it requires minimal equipment and can be initiated immediately at the onset of arrest. In clinical practice, the intent is that BLS will be performed in conjunction with ALS and appropriate monitoring as possible.

BASIC LIFE SUPPORT

Key points
- Recognize the need for CPR
- Rapidly start CPR
- Start ventilation at a rate of 10 bpm
- Start chest compressions at a rate of at least 100 bpm
- Change person doing the chest compressions every 2 minutes, if possible

The first thing to do is to evaluate if the foal is suitable for CPR. Not all foals are suitable candidates for resuscitation. Foals with obvious congenital defects at birth should probably not be resuscitated. The welfare and financial implications of resuscitation should always be considered.

What to Do

- Patient positioning
- Ensure adequate airway (intubation is possible)
- Start ventilation
- Evaluate need for circulatory support
- Start chest compressions if required

Patient Positioning

Place the foal in lateral recumbency on a hard, flat surface. If you can, quickly check if the foal has any fractured ribs. If these are found, place the side with the fractured ribs against the ground, and in case of bilaterally fractured ribs, place the side with more of the cranial ribs (3, 4, and 5) fractured on the ground.

Ventilation

The best way to ensure an adequate airway is to intubate the foal. Intubation via the nose is preferred to intubation via the mouth to prevent the foal chewing the tube when it regains consciousness. However, as time is of the essence only 2 quick attempts should be used for nasotracheal intubation after which the oral route should be used. A 55-cm long cuffed endotracheal tube is recommended. The diameter of the tube should be matched with the size of the foal and be as large as possible to decrease the resistance to flow. As a rough rule, a 9 to 10 mm tube fits most newborn thoroughbred foals, whereas large warm bloods may need tubes as large as 10 to 12 mm. On the other hand, Arabian and pony foals may need smaller tubes.

Ideally sterile technique should be used to avoid introduction of nosocomial pathogens; however, first priority is rapid intubation and initiation of resuscitation. It is important to extend the head so that it is in a straight line with the neck. To pass the tube via the nose, push the tube ventrally toward the ventral meatus medially with one hand while gently advancing the tube with the other hand. When passing the tube via the mouth, the tongue should be pulled forward and slightly lateral with one hand to stabilize the larynx. The tube is advanced in the midline over the tongue. In both cases, the tube should be rotated or twisted once reaching the larynx. When the tube reaches the larynx one helpful tip is also to stabilize the larynx with the other hand externally while advancing the tube to facilitate the correct positioning. The endotracheal tube should be advanced until only the adapter is visible at the nostril to minimize the dead space. Once the tube is in place the cuff is inflated. It is also wise to secure the tube in place with bandage material around the head, muzzle, or bottom jaw.

It is usually not difficult to ensure that the tube is in the trachea. One can compress the chest and feel for the expired air. Also, the chest wall should rise when the breaths are being given. On the other hand, if the tube has been placed in the esophagus it can usually be felt in the cranial neck dorsal to the proximal trachea.

When an endotracheal tube is not immediately available, ventilation with a pump and mask or mouth-to-nose ventilation can be effective. The fact that foals are obligate nasal breathers makes these methods relatively effective. For both methods, the head and neck should be maximally extended to reduce the risk of aerophagia. Aerophagia fills the stomach with gas and can prevent the lungs from fully expanding. For mouth-to-nose resuscitation, the opposite nostril should be held closed. While blowing into the nostril or pushing the pump, one should observe the chest rising, ensuring that the air is reaching the lungs and that the tidal volume is adequate.

RECOVER Recommendations for Ventilation

1. Inspiratory time: 1-s inspiratory time with long expiratory time—short, infrequent breaths recommended.
2. Ventilation rate: based on porcine studies a ventilation rate of 10 breaths/min is recommended and target is to achieve normocapnia while avoiding arterial hypoxemia.[17–20]
3. Tidal volume: 10 mL/kg
4. Room air instead of 100% oxygen[21,22]

The optimum rate of ventilation is suggested to be around 10 to 20 breaths/min. Increased thoracic pressure induced by positive-pressure ventilation can interfere significantly with cardiac return and decreases coronary and cerebral perfusion. Human infant and experimental animal evidence suggests decreased neurologic injury when oxygen supplementation is titrated to achieve normoxemia (PaO_2 of 80–105 mm Hg) compared with animals that are hyperoxemic. This is why an FiO_2 of 21% (room air) during CPR of human newborns is recommended.[21,22] The best method of providing artificial respiration is a self-inflating bag-valve device designed for human adult resuscitation (1600 mL bag) connected to an endotracheal tube. This device allows controlled ventilation and avoids the risk of aerophagia, or forcing material (such as meconium or mucus) into the airways. When using a resuscitation bag, the bag can either be placed between the hands and squeezed or on the floor and pushed empty with both hands placed flat and together over the bag.

Thoracic Compressions

The foal should be reassessed 30 seconds after starting the ventilation. Thoracic compressions should be started if the heartbeat is absent, less than 40 bpm, or less than 50 bpm and not increasing. The person performing the thoracic compressions should kneel parallel to the foal's spine and place his or her hands on top of each other, just caudal to the foal's triceps, at the highest point of the thorax. The shoulders should be directly above the hands, enabling use of the body weight to help compress the thorax. This helps to deliver enough force and also to reduce resuscitator fatigue.

In rare cases of witnessed arrest of presumed primary cardiac origin, the immediate provision of thoracic compressions should be the priority. Based on the fact that most cardiac arrests in foals are secondary to respiratory arrest and the ease of foal intubation, prolonged thoracic-compression-only CPR is not recommended and intubation and ventilation should be attempted as soon as possible, while compressions are being performed.

Increased depth of compression was associated with an increased rate of successful defibrillation and ROSC in human patients and in pig models.[23–30]

RECOVER Recommendations

- Optimal compression depth can be achieved by "pushing hard"
- Continuous thoracic compressions should be performed if there is more than 1 resuscitator. No pauses should be made
- Compression to ventilation (CV) ratio of 30:2
- Thoracic compression rate 100 to 120 bpm

The optimal compression depth in lateral recumbency in dogs and cats has not been examined, but a compression depth of between one-third and half the width of the thorax is reasonable. It would appear that the current human recommendation to "push hard" is likely to be applicable to veterinary medicine.

In experimental pig studies, it has been shown that it takes approximately 60 seconds of continuous thoracic compressions to build up maximal coronary perfusion pressure (CPP) and pauses in thoracic compressions are associated with immediate decreases in CPP.[31,32]

A porcine study comparing continuous thoracic compressions without ventilation to CPR with a C:V ratio of 30:2 in pigs found no difference in hemodynamic performance but cerebral oxygen delivery was improved when the pigs were also ventilated.[33] Continuous thoracic compressions or a C:V ratio of 100:2 had lower rates of ROSC and poorer blood gas parameters compared with the 30:2 or 100:5 groups in another porcine study.[34]

Recommendation

For single-rescuer CPR without the patient being intubated, a C:V ratio of 30:2 is currently recommended, but continuous thoracic compressions should be performed for intubated patients.

Thoracic compressions aim to generate blood flow to vital organs during CPR. Ideal thoracic compressions may achieve a cardiac output of approximately 25% to 30% of normal, at most. An adult horse study showed that compression rates of 80 bpm were superior to either 60 or 40 bpm in terms of blood flow achieved.[35] Both canine[36,37] and human studies have shown that higher compression rates (100–120/min vs 60/min) are associated with far better survival rates.

Overall there is evidence to support that interposed abdominal compression (IAC) CPR may be superior to standard CPR and is unlikely to cause harm. It is important to note that many studies used automated devices to perform IAC-CPR, so the ability to generate similar results in clinical veterinary patients using manual techniques is unknown.

ADVANCED LIFE SUPPORT

ALS includes therapy with vasopressors, positive inotropes, anticholinergics, correction of electrolyte disturbances, volume deficits, severe anemia, and prompt defibrillation. It should be noted that with the exception of defibrillation, it is controversial as to whether ALS improves long-term outcomes.

Key points
- Standard dose epinephrine is the drug of choice for CPR
- Rapid defibrillation is warranted in animals with observed progression to ventricular tachycardia (VT) or VF
- Defibrillation should follow a cycle of CPR in unwitnessed pulseless VT or VF
- Open chest CPR might be considered in select cases with access to post-cardiac arrest support
- Reversal of anesthetic agents and corrections of major acid-base and electrolyte disturbances is advisable

Vasopressor and Vagolytic Therapy

Epinephrine dose

Epinephrine is the principal drug for resuscitation of the foal, although recent human studies have questioned its effect.[38] The recommended dose has not changed and is 0.01 mg/kg IV every 3 to 5 minutes. Increased doses have been researched but human and porcine studies suggest high-dose epinephrine (0.1 mg/kg) might have harmful effects.[39–43] No studies have been published on small animals or horses.

Vasopressin Versus Epinephrine

Porcine models show a beneficial effect of using either vasopressin alone or in combination with epinephrine.[44–46] Human studies show no consistent benefit. One dog study showed no difference in ROSC between dogs receiving vasopressin or epinephrine.[47] No studies in horses have been published.

Atropine

Atropine is most likely harmless but there is no strong evidence supporting its use in any species and it should not be used.

Defibrillation

Current guidelines in human medicine have switched from airway—breathing—circulation to the prompt use of defibrillation first due to the high incidence of shockable rhythms (ie, VF or pulseless VT) in humans. As previously noted this is not the case in horses. However, electrical defibrillation may be attempted in a foal in asystole that does not respond to chest compressions and epinephrine injection.

Defibrillator paste is applied to the paddles. Paddles are placed firmly on opposite sides of the thorax at the level of the costochondral junction. In foals in lateral recumbency, a posterior paddle is placed on the down side and the hand paddle on the up side. Once the machine is set, the person using the defibrillator announces an audible "clear" and visually ensures all personnel including the one providing the shock are not in contact with the table or the patient. One single shock is provided after which chest compressions and ventilation should immediately resume. ECG should only be evaluated after one cardiac compression cycle (2 minutes) is complete and then determine if a second defibrillation is necessary. The dose is 2 to 4 J/kg (100–200 J/50 kg foal), increasing the energy by 50% with each defibrillation attempt.

Defibrillation Technique

There are 2 types of electric defibrillators available, mono- and biphasic. Biphasic has become standard in human medicine as it requires less energy. Single-shock method should be used as it enables less interruption to chest compressions reducing myocardial ischemia. No study investigating either one of these has been performed in small animals or horses. Studies suggest that if CPA is prolonged and lasted more than 4 minutes, CPR should be performed first. In veterinary medicine in clinical settings neither the duration of CPA nor the character of the possible cardiac arrhythmia are known making recommendations less clear.

When using high frequencies for defibrillation, the risk of myocardial damage increases equally. However, not using high enough frequencies results in patient death. For monophasic defibrillators, increasing energy doses are associated with increased defibrillation success in animals in which defibrillation at a lower dose failed. Current human literature is in favor of escalating dosage protocol and the same should apply to animals.

Antiarrhythmic Drug Therapy

In small animals, rapid defibrillation or cardioversion is advised before drug therapy, and in fact worse outcomes with the use of antiarrhythmic drugs during CPR have been reported in people.[48,49] The conclusion is that only in VF that is resistant to shock therapy may amiodarone be helpful. No role for other antiarrhythmic agents including lidocaine, bretylium or magnesium has been proved.

Electrolyte Therapy

The advantage of monitoring electrolyte concentrations during CPR has been investigated. Little evidence exists to promote the monitoring of electrolytes except for potassium. Potassium is released from cells during ischemia, and increased potassium concentrations can be used as a prognostic factor. Hemodialysis could be used to decrease the potassium concentration below 8 mmol/L to improve resuscitation results.[50–53] Calcium use has been suggested in cases of calcium channel blocker overdose, severe hypocalcemia, and hyperkalemia to improve cardiac function.

Other Therapies

Corticosteroid administration has no proven beneficial effect and a possible harmful effect, so presently its use is not recommended in CPR. Low-dose corticosteroid treatment of patients with persistent hypotension requiring sympathomimetic support may be considered in the post–cardiac-arrest period.

Impedance threshold devices (ITDs) use the interdependence of the respiratory and circulatory systems to create a negative pressure within the thorax during the CPR release phase, resulting in enhanced venous return during CPR. Some porcine models also suggest that this can lead to reductions in intracranial pressure, which could theoretically improve cerebral perfusion during CPR.[54] No negative effects of an ITD have been observed in experimental animals. Several human studies have demonstrated that the use of an ITD was associated with a higher ROSC and short-term survival, and some studies have found improvements in long-term survival.[55–57] Veterinary medicine clinical studies are lacking.

Sodium bicarbonate administration to correct academia in animals requiring CPA has been proposed. Acidemia can impair the effect of catecholamines on vasculature. However, the risks of administering bicarbonate include increase in serum osmolarity and alkalemia potentially resulting in paradoxic cerebral and metabolic acidosis. Studies show conflicting results, which seem to depend on the duration of cardiac arrest and timing of buffer administration. At the moment, routine use of sodium bicarbonate in CPA is not recommended.

Intratracheal Drug Administration

Drugs that could be given via intratracheal (IT) administration include epinephrine, vasopressin, and atropine. The absorption of these drugs has been shown to be effective during anesthesia[58–61] but the absorption during CPA is unknown. If given IT, the use of epinephrine should be increased 10-fold. These drugs should be diluted in ideally sterile water or if not available, saline and delivered via a catheter to at least the level of carina and ideally further down in the tracheal tree. There are no human studies showing adult survivors of IT-only CPR, and in infants IT CPR is recommended only as a short-term solution when immediate intravenous access is not a possibility.

Open Chest CPR

In cases of significant intrathoracic disease, such as penetrating injuries, tension pneumothorax, or pericardial effusion, it may be beneficial to perform open chest instead of standard CPR. Aftercare is challenging and a defibrillator should be readily available. Aseptic technique is of utmost importance. De Moor and colleagues[62] described 2 cases, 1 pony and 1 horse, using intrathoracic cardiac resuscitation. Both responded initially but the pony died immediately after resuscitation due to traumatic head injury and the horse died 10 days after resuscitation due to massive intrathoracic infection.

MONITORING

Key points
- Time spent verifying an absent pulse may delay onset of CPR
- ECG analysis of an unresponsive patient may be used to identify arrhythmias requiring specific treatment
- Pauses in chest compressions to evaluate the ECG should be minimized
- $EtCO_2$ monitoring is useful to identify ROSC and may be prognostic
- Monitoring after CPR should be tailored to each patient

Monitoring Patients During CPA

Verification of CPA by palpation of peripheral pulses is not reliable, even though loss of peripheral pulse pressure may precede cardiac arrest in CPA and could be used to predict incoming CPA. Continuous Doppler monitoring is not practical clinically, especially in horses, and so these would only rarely be placed beforehand.

The use of ECG to diagnose CPA must be done with caution as pulseless electrical activity can be mistaken for a perfusing rhythm. ECG analysis does enable the identification of rhythms that can be treated with defibrillation (eg, VF). On the other hand, ECG can be used to rule out CPA in patients with syncope or collapse.

The correlation between $EtCO_2$ and cardiac output is a useful way to diagnose CPA in ventilated animals because a sudden decrease in $EtCO_2$ level is highly suggestive of CPA. However, in nonventilated animals, the $EtCO_2$ can behave variably and thus cannot be used on its own. Confirmation of endotracheal tube placement can be done with $EtCO_2$. A high value for $EtCO_2$ would confirm placement in the trachea as the concentration is usually very low in the stomach and esophagus. However, if $EtCO_2$ is low, it is still possible that the tube is correctly placed, and therefore it is best to also use clinical assessment to confirm correct placement such as chest wall movement, direct visualization of the endotracheal tube between the arytenoid cartilages, auscultation of air movement in hemithoraces, or the presence of condensation on the inside of the endotracheal tube. One practical problem with monitoring $EtCO_2$ in newborn foals is that the large amount of fluid that comes out of the lungs can interfere with the $EtCO_2$ monitoring equipment.

One of the questions arising from RECOVER was whether blood gas monitoring would improve and/or predict outcome in animals being resuscitated. There is only one veterinary study available providing information on prognostic indicators for CPA in dogs and cats undergoing nonexperimental arrests.[2] The mean highest recorded $EtCO_2$ was significantly higher in dogs that achieved ROSC (36.6 ± 19.7 mm Hg) than those that did not (10.3 ± 10.2 mm Hg). Similar was reported by Kern and colleagues,[63,64] where a decline in $EtCO_2$ was seen during CPR in the dogs in which ROSC was not obtained, whereas $EtCO_2$ remained constant in the dogs that were successfully resuscitated. On the other hand, $EtCO_2$ can also be used to diagnose ROSC during resuscitation. Chalak and colleagues[65] reported that $EtCO_2$ concentration increased rapidly when ROSC was achieved and that a value of 14 mm Hg had a sensitivity of 93% and a specificity of 81% for prediction of the presence of an audible heartbeat in piglets. These piglets underwent CPR with continuous $EtCO_2$ monitoring, and cardiac auscultation was performed every 30 seconds.

The effect of monitoring ventilatory parameters during resuscitation is unknown. It is a common mistake to ventilate too frequently, even among experienced personnel. Ventilatory rates higher than 10 to 12 breaths/min should be avoided for 2 reasons: first, time spent without cardiac compressions in single-rescuer scenarios should be minimized and second, increased time with positive intrathoracic pressure will have a negative effect on hemodynamics. However, optimal ventilation rates are unknown, and thus it was suggested that monitoring ventilatory parameters would be beneficial.[66–68]

Controversy in monitoring blood gas parameters during CPR lies in the delay of changes in these values in the early stages of CPA. One of the questions regarding the use of these values during CPR is whether the sample should be arterial or venous. A couple of veterinary studies have been performed. Sato and colleagues[69] evaluated the association between arteriovenous difference in the partial pressure of CO_2 (PCO_2) and cardiac output during CPR in dogs. The results show that mixed venous PCO_2 and pH was better associated with low cardiac output states than arterial values. This was in agreement with a previous study that noted mixed venous blood gas values changing to a greater degree during the resuscitation period than the arterial samples.[70,71] Similar results have been reported in a swine CPA model.[72]

The use of ECG analysis to predict defibrillation success has been investigated in people. Based on laboratory investigations in dogs and swine, coarse VF is more likely to respond with ROSC following defibrillation than fine VF. However, waveform analysis that can predict defibrillation success has not been determined and cannot be used as a prognostic factor.

When to Stop

Ventilation should be stopped when the heart rate is greater than 60 bpm and spontaneous breathing is well established; this can be tested by stopping ventilation and disconnecting the bag or pump for 30 seconds. The first few breaths may be gasping but after these the foal should have a respiratory rate greater than 16 breaths/min, a regular respiratory pattern, and normal respiratory effort. Premature withdrawal of ventilation is reported to be the most common mistake in human neonatal CPR.

Chest compressions should be continued until a regular heartbeat of more than 60 bpm has been established. There should be no lag period between the stopping of support and the onset of a spontaneous heartbeat. When testing for adequacy of heart beat, CPR should not be stopped for longer than 10 seconds at a time. Clinical experience suggests that if spontaneous circulation and respiration are not present after 10 minutes, then survival is unlikely.

POST–CARDIAC ARREST CARE

Key points
- Organ perfusion should be optimized with fluid therapy and possibly inotropes and vasopressors
- Aim for normoxemia, not hyperoxemia
- Mild hypothermia may be beneficial in the early post-resuscitation period
- There is no evidence to support routine administration of corticosteroids, antiseizure prophylaxis, mannitol, or metabolic protectants after cardiac arrest.

Human studies suggest that early correction to optimize hemodynamic variables have a beneficial effect. However, further studies are required and no optimal target end-points have been determined. Interventions included in these human protocols were fluid and pressor administration guided by central venous oxygen saturation ($ScvO_2$), blood lactate, and central venous and arterial blood pressure.

Myocardial stunning (a reversible phenomenon that happens early after global myocardial ischemia in which left and right ventricular ejection fractions decrease and end diastolic pressure increases) may contribute to the hemodynamic dysfunction. Patients suffering form this generally respond to inotropic therapy. Both Herlitz and colleagues[73] and Trzeciak and colleagues[74] have reported a correlation between hypotension after resuscitation from cardiac arrest and decreased survival and neurologic outcome, indicating the importance of the avoidance of hypotension in the PCA period.

The goal of PCA care is to avoid hypotension and maintain adequate perfusion to the tissues. However, perfusion depends on blood flow not blood pressure alone, and thus it is advisable to not only monitor blood pressure but also to measure global perfusion metrics such as $ScvO_2$ and blood lactate.

The general agreement is that intravenous fluids are beneficial in the post-resuscitation period to maintain and/or achieve normal blood flow. However, no consensus has been reached as to the type and volume of fluids that would be optimal. Again despite associated better outcomes with cardioactive/vasopressor therapy for PCA hypotension in some studies, no definitive beneficial evidence exists.

The preponderance of evidence from clinical human and experimental canine studies suggest a beneficial effect on neurologic intact survival if mild hypothermia (core temperature of $33°C \pm 1°C$) is instituted as soon as possible and maintained for more than 12 hours. Although the evidence is lacking with respect to specific rates of rewarming after accidental or therapeutic hypothermia, slower rewarming rates appear to be preferred over faster ones in several related populations and evaluated endpoints.

Cerebral edema after cardiac arrest has been described in people, and its occurrence appears to be correlated with poor outcome.[75,76] Both mannitol and hypertonic saline have been recommended in dogs and cats if cerebral edema or elevated intracranial hypertension is suspected.[77,78] Hypertonic saline should not be used in neonatal foals as they cannot handle rapid changes in sodium.

RESUSCITATION AT THE TIME OF FOALING

Resuscitation at the time of birth is a special case of CPR in equine neonates. Compared with older neonates requiring CPR, these foals carry a better prognosis for both ROSC and survival to discharge. However, rapid intervention is often needed, and therefore, it is important to recognize mares whose foals are at increased risk beforehand so that preparations can be made. Risk factors during pregnancy include any maternal disease such as placentitis (vaginal discharge during pregnancy, uteroplacental thickening) or any other systemic disease of the dam, dystocia, or cesarean section.

The resuscitation itself follows the same principles as previously described. In the newborn foal, the airways need to be cleared of membranes. Also, vigorous towel drying should be started immediately as it acts as a strong stimulus to the foal to start breathing. In a foal that is born with meconium staining, the first 20 seconds should be devoted to suctioning fluids from the airway. Airway suctioning should ideally start as soon as a meconium-stained head appears at the vulva, before the foal takes its first breath. This early suctioning is clearly not always possible. If the foal is covered in thick meconium, suctioning of fluids from the trachea should also be attempted. Suctioning of fluids from the oropharynx can induce bradycardia or even cardiac arrest via vagal reflexes, and for this reason, suctioning with a bulb syringe may be safer than using a mechanical unit. Mechanical suction should not be applied for longer than 5 to 10 seconds at a time.

SUMMARY

In selected cases, resuscitation of the foal can be a worthwhile procedure, with good outcomes. This is especially the case in newborn foals that arrest as a consequence of the birthing procedure, rather than due to an intercurrent disease. The RECOVER initiative has not only benefited small animals but has also allowed us to focus on what is presumed current best practice in foals based on data and research from other species. Moreover, it has again highlighted the large knowledge gaps that surround resuscitation of the neonatal foal.

REFERENCES

1. Boller M, Fletcher DJ. RECOVER evidence and knowledge gap analysis on veterinary CPR. Part 1: evidence analysis and consensus process: collaborative path toward small animal CPR guidelines. J Vet Emerg Crit Care (San Antonio) 2012;22(Suppl 1):S4–12. http://dx.doi.org/10.1111/j.1476-4431.2012.00758.x.
2. Hofmeister EH, Brainard BM, Egger CM, et al. Prognostic indicators for dogs and cats with cardiopulmonary arrest treated by cardiopulmonary cerebral resuscitation at a university teaching hospital. J Am Vet Med Assoc 2009;235:50–7.
3. Hopper K, Epstein SE, Fletcher DJ, et al, RECOVER Basic Life Support Domain Authors. RECOVER evidence and knowledge gap analysis on veterinary CPR. Part 3: basic life support. J Vet Emerg Crit Care (San Antonio) 2012;22(Suppl 1):S26–43. http://dx.doi.org/10.1111/j.1476-4431.2012.00753.x.
4. Kass PH, Haskins SC. Survival following cardiopulmonary resuscitation in dogs and cats. J Vet Emerg Crit Care 1992;2:57–65.
5. Wingfield WE, Van Pelt DR. Respiratory and cardiopulmonary ar- rest in dogs and cats: 265 cases (1986–1991). J Am Vet Med Assoc 1992;200:1993–6.
6. Meaney PA, Nadkarni VM, Kern KB, et al. Rhythms and outcomes of adult in-hospital cardiac arrest. Crit Care Med 2010;38:101–8.
7. Peberdy MA, Kaye W, Ornato JP, et al. Cardiopulmonary resuscitation of adults in the hospital: a report of 14720 cardiac arrests from the National Registry of Cardiopulmonary Resuscitation. Resuscitation 2003;58:297–308.
8. Frauenfelder HC. External cardiovascular resuscitation of the anesthetized pony. J Am Vet Med Assoc 1981;179:673–6.
9. Palmer JE. VETTalks on cutting-edge research in critical care: CPR case series IVECCS. Proceedings. 2013.
10. Palmer JE. Neonatal foal resuscitation. Vet Clin North Am Equine Pract 2007;23: 159–82.
11. Eisenberg MS. Incidence and significance of gasping or agonal respirations in cardiac arrest patients. Curr Opin Crit Care 2006;12(3):204–6.
12. White L, Rogers J, Bloomingdale M, et al. Dispatcher-assisted cardiopulmonary resuscitation: risks for patients not in cardiac arrest. Circulation 2010;121(1): 91–7.
13. McCue PM, Ferris RA. Parturition, dystocia and foal survival: A retrospective study of 1047 births. Equine Vet J Suppl 2012;(41):22–5.
14. McMichael M, Herring J, Fletcher DJ, et al, RECOVER Preparedness and Prevention Domain Worksheet Authors. RECOVER evidence and knowledge gap analysis on veterinary CPR. Part 2: preparedness and prevention. J Vet Emerg Crit Care 2012;22(Suppl 1):S13–25. http://dx.doi.org/10.1111/j.1476-4431.2012.00752.x.
15. Yamamoto K, Yasuda J, Too K, et al. Arrhythmias in newborn thoroughbred foals. Equine Vet J 1992;24(3):169–73.
16. Aufderheide TP, Yannopoulos D, Lick CJ, et al. Implementing the 2005 American Heart Association Guidelines improves outcomes after out-of-hospital cardiac arrest. Heart Rhythm 2010;7(10):1357–62.

17. Cavus E, Meybohm P, Bein B, et al. Impact of different compression-ventilation ratios during basic life support cardiopulmonary resuscitation. Resuscitation 2008;79(1):118–24.

18. Lurie KG, Yannopoulos D, McKnite SH, et al. Comparison of a 10- breaths-per-minute versus a 2-breaths-per-minute strategy during cardiopulmonary resuscitation in a porcine model of cardiac arrest. Respir Care 2008;53(7):862–70.

19. Yannopoulos D, Matsuura T, McKnite S, et al. No assisted ventilation cardiopulmonary resuscitation and 24-hour neurological outcomes in a porcine model of cardiac arrest. Crit Care Med 2010;38(1):254–60.

20. Yannopoulos D, Sigurdsson G, McKnite S, et al. Reducing venti- lation frequency combined with an inspiratory impedance device improves CPR efficiency in swine model of cardiac arrest. Resuscitation 2004;61(1):75–82.

21. Saugstad OD, Rootwelt T, Aalen O. Resuscitation of asphyxiated newborn infants with room air or oxygen: an international controlled trial: the Resair 2 study. Pediatrics 1998;102(1):e1.

22. Saugstad OD, Vento M, Ramji S, et al. Neurodevelopmental outcome of infants resuscitated with air or 100% oxygen: a systematic review and meta-analysis. Neonatology 2012;102(2):98–103.

23. Babbs CF, Kemeny AE, Quan W, et al. A new paradigm for human resuscitation research using intelligent devices. Resuscitation 2008;77(3):306–15.

24. Balan IS, Fiskum G, Hazelton J, et al. Oximetry-guided reoxygena- tion improves neurological outcome after experimental cardiac arrest. Stroke 2006;37(12): 3008–13.

25. Bohn A, Weber TP, Wecker S, et al. The addition of voice prompts to audiovisual feedback and debriefing does not modify CPR quality or outcomes in out of hospital cardiac arrest–a prospective, randomized trial. Resuscitation 2011;82(3): 257–62.

26. Edelson DP, Abella BS, Kramer-Johansen J, et al. Effects of com- pression depth and pre-shock pauses predict defibrillation failure during cardiac arrest. Resuscitation 2006;71(2):137–45.

27. Kramer-Johansen J, Myklebust H, Wik L, et al. Quality of out-of- hospital cardiopulmonary resuscitation with real time automated feedback: a prospective interventional study. Resuscitation 2006;71(3):283–92.

28. Li Y, Ristagno G, Bisera J, et al. Electrocardiogram waveforms for monitoring effectiveness of chest compression during cardiopul- monary resuscitation. Crit Care Med 2008;36(1):211–5.

29. Ristagno G, Tang W, Chang YT, et al. The quality of chest compres- sions during cardiopulmonary resuscitation overrides importance of timing of defibrillation. Chest 2007;132(1):70–5.

30. Rozanski EA, Rush JE, Buckley GJ, et al. RECOVER evidence and knowledge gap analysis on veterinary CPR. Part 4: advanced life support. J Vet Emerg Crit Care (San Antonio) 2012;22(Suppl 1):S44–64. http://dx.doi.org/10.1111/j. 1476-4431.2012.00755.x.

31. Berg RA, Sanders AB, Kern KB, et al. Adverse hemodynamic effects of interrupting chest compressions for rescue breathing dur- ing cardiopulmonary resuscitation for ventricular fibrillation car- diac arrest. Circulation 2001;104(20):2465–70.

32. Kern KB, Hilwig RW, Berg RA, et al. Efficacy of chest compression-only BLS CPR in the presence of an occluded airway. Resuscitation 1998;39(3):179–88.

33. Dorph E, Wik L, Strømme TA, et al. Oxygen delivery and return of spontaneous circulation with ventilation:compression ratio 2:30 versus chest compressions only CPR in pigs. Resuscitation 2004;60(3):309–18.

34. Kill C, Torossian A, Freisburger C, et al. Basic life support with four different compression/ventilation ratios in a pig model: the need for ventilation. Resuscitation 2009;80(9):1060–5.

35. Hubbell JA, Muir WW, Gaynor JS. Cardiovascular effects of thoracic compression in horses subjected to euthanasia. Equine Vet J 1993;25(4):282–4.

36. Feneley MP, Maier GW, Kern KB, et al. Influence of compression rate on initial success of resuscitation and 24 hour survival after prolonged manual cardiopulmonary resuscitation in dogs. Circulation 1988;77(1):240–50.

37. Fletcher DJ, Brainard BM, Boller M, et al. RECOVER evidence and knowledge gap analysis on veterinary CPR. Part 7: clinical guidelines. J Vet Emerg Crit Care (San Antonio) 2012;22(Suppl 1):S102–31. http://dx.doi.org/10.1111/j.1476-4431.2012.00757.x.

38. Jacobs IG, Finn JC, Jelinek GA, et al. Effect of adrenaline on survival in out-of-hospital cardiac arrest: a randomised double-blind placebo-controlled trial. Resuscitation 2011;82(9):1138–43.

39. Berg RA, Otto CW, Kern KB, et al. A randomized, blinded trial of high-dose epinephrine versus standard-dose epinephrine in a swine model of pediatric asphyxial cardiac arrest. Crit Care Med 1996;24(10):1695–700.

40. Berg RA, Otto CW, Kern KB, et al. High-dose epinephrine results in greater early mortality after resuscitation from prolonged cardiac arrest in pigs: a prospective, randomized study. Crit Care Med 1994;22(2):282–90.

41. Stiell IG, Hebert PC, Weitzman BN, et al. High-dose epinephrine in adult cardiac arrest. N Engl J Med 1992;327(15):1045–50.

42. Vandycke C, Martens P. High dose versus standard doseepinephrine in cardiac arrest - a meta-analysis. Resuscitation 2000;45(3):161–6.

43. Woodhouse SP, Cox S, Boyd P, et al. High dose and standard dose adrenaline do not alter survival, compared with placebo, incardiac arrest. Resuscitation 1995;30(3):243–9.

44. Stadlbauer KH, Wagner-Berger HG, Wenzel V, et al. Survival with full neurologic recovery after prolonged cardiopulmonary resuscitation with a combination of vasopressin and epinephrine in pigs. Anesth Analg 2003;96(6):1743–9 [table of contents].

45. Smarick SD, Haskins SC, Boller M, et al. RECOVER evidence and knowledge gap analysis on veterinary CPR. Part 6: post-cardiac arrest care. J Vet Emerg Crit Care (San Antonio) 2012;22(Suppl 1):S85–101. http://dx.doi.org/10.1111/j.1476-4431.2012.00754.x.

46. Wenzel V, Lindner KH, Krismer AC, et al. Survival with full neurologic recovery and no cerebral pathology after prolonged car- diopulmonary resuscitation with vasopressin in pigs. J Am Coll Cardiol 2000;35(2):527–33.

47. Buckley GJ, Rozanski EA, Rush JE. Randomized, blinded com- parison of epinephrine and vasopressin for treatment of naturally occurring cardiopulmonary arrest in dogs. J Vet Intern Med 2011;25(6):1334–40.

48. Frame LH. The effect of chronic oral and acute intravenous amiodarone administration on ventricular defibrillation threshold using implanted electrodes in dogs. Pacing Clin Electrophysiol 1989;12(2):339–46.

49. Markel DT, Gold LS, Allen J, et al. Procainamide and survival in ventricular fibrillation out-of-hospital cardiac arrest. Acad Emerg Med 2010;17(6):617–23.

50. Bender PR, Debehnke DJ, Swart GL, et al. Serum potassium con- centration as a predictor of resuscitation outcome in hypothermic cardiac arrest. Wilderness Environ Med 1995;6(3):273–82.

51. Engoren M, Severyn F, Fenn-Buderer N, et al. Cardiac output, coronary blood flow, and blood gases during open-chest standard and compression-active-decompression cardiopulmonary resuscitation. Resuscitation 2002;55(3):309–16.
52. Lin JL, Lim PS, Leu ML, et al. Outcomes of severe hyperkalemia in cardiopulmonary resuscitation with concomitant hemodialysis. Intensive Care Med 1994;20(4):287–90.
53. Niemann JT, Cairns CB. Hyperkalemia and ionized hypocalcemia during cardiac arrest and resuscitation: possible culprits for post- countershock arrhythmias? Ann Emerg Med 1999;34(1):1–7.
54. Yannopoulos D, Aufderheide TP, McKnite S, et al. Hemodynamic and respiratory effects of negative tracheal pressure during CPR in pigs. Resuscitation 2006;69(3):487–94.
55. Aufderheide TP, Pirrallo RG, Provo TA, et al. Clinical evaluation of an inspiratory impedance threshold device during standard car- diopulmonary resuscitation in patients with out-of-hospital cardiac arrest. Crit Care Med 2005;33(4):734–40.
56. Plaisance P, Lurie KG, Vicaut E, et al. Evaluation of an impedance threshold device in patients receiving active compression– decompression cardiopulmonary resuscitation for out of hospital cardiac arrest. Resuscitation 2004;61(3):265–71.
57. Thigpen K, Davis SP, Basol R, et al. Implementing the 2005 American Heart Association guidelines, including use of the impedance threshold device, improves hospital discharge rate after in-hospital cardiac arrest. Respir Care 2010;55(8):1014–9.
58. Efrati O, Barak A, Ben-Abraham R, et al. Hemodynamic effects of tracheal administration of vasopressin in dogs. Resuscitation 2001;50(2):227–32.
59. Kleinman ME, Oh W, Stonestreet BS. Comparison of intravenous and endotracheal epinephrine during cardiopulmonary resuscitation in newborn piglets. Crit Care Med 1999;27(12):2748–54.
60. Manisterski Y, Vaknin Z, Ben-Abraham R, et al. Endotracheal epinephrine: a call for larger doses. Anesth Analg 2002;95(4):1037–41 [table of contents].
61. Paret G, Mazkereth R, Sella R, et al. Atropine pharmacokinetics and pharmacodynamics following endotracheal versus endobronchial administration in dogs. Resuscitation 1999;41(1):57–62.
62. De Moor A, Verschooten F, Desmet P, et al. Intrathoracic cardiac resuscitation in the horse. Equine Vet J 1972;4:31–3.
63. Kern KB, Sanders AB, Voorhees WD, et al. Changes in expired end-tidal carbon dioxide during cardiopulmonary resuscitation in dogs: a prognostic guide for resuscitation efforts. J Am Coll Cardiol 1989;13(5):1184–9.
64. Kilgannon JH, Roberts BW, Reihl LR, et al. Early arterial hypoten- sion is common in the post-cardiac arrest syndrome and associated with increased in-hospital mortality. Resuscitation 2008;79(3):410–6.
65. Chalak LF, Barber CA, Hynan L, et al. End-tidal CO2 detection of an audible heart rate during neonatal cardiopulmonary resuscitation after asystole in asphyxiated piglets. Pediatr Res 2011;69(5 Pt 1):401–5.
66. Brainard BM, Boller M, Fletcher DJ, et al. RECOVER evidence and knowledge gap analysis on veterinary CPR. Part 5: monitoring. J Vet Emerg Crit Care (San Antonio) 2012;22(Suppl 1):S65–84. http://dx.doi.org/10.1111/j.1476-4431.2012.00751.x.
67. Brodbelt DC, Blissitt KJ, Hammond RA, et al. The risk of death: the confidential enquiry into perioperative small animal fatalities. Vet Anaesth Analg 2008;35(5):365–73.

68. Brücken A, Kaab AB, Kottmann K, et al. Reducing the duration of 100% oxygen ventilation in the early reperfusion period after cardiopulmonary resuscitation decreases striatal brain damage. Resuscitation 2010;81(12):1698–703.

69. Sato S, Okubo N, Satsumae T, et al. Arteriovenous differences in PCO2 and cardiac output during CPR in the dog. Resuscitation 1994;27(3):255–9.

70. Ralston SH, Voorhees WD, Showen L, et al. Venous and arterial blood gases during and after cardiopulmonary resuscitation in dogs. Am J Emerg Med 1985;3(2):132–6.

71. Reynolds JC, Rittenberger JC, Menegazzi JJ. Drug administration in animal studies of cardiac arrest does not reflect human clinical experience. Resuscitation 2007;74(1):13–26.

72. Tucker KJ, Idris AH, Wenzel V, et al. Changes in arterial and mixed venous blood gases during untreated ventricular fibrillation and cardiopulmonary resuscitation. Resuscitation 1994;28(2):137–41.

73. Herlitz J, Ekström L, Wennerblom B, et al. Hospital mortality after out-of-hospital cardiac arrest among patients found in ventricular fibrillation. Resuscitation 1995;29(1):11–21.

74. Trzeciak S, Jones AE, Kilgannon JH, et al. Significance of arterial hypotension after resuscitation from cardiac arrest. Crit Care Med 2009;37(11):2895–903 [quiz: 2904].

75. Metter RB, Rittenberger JC, Guyette FX, et al. Association between a quantitative CT scan measure of brain edema and outcome after cardiac arrest. Resuscitation 2011;82(9):1180–5.

76. Wright WL, Geocadin RG. Postresuscitative intensive care: neu- roprotective strategies after cardiac arrest. Semin Neurol 2006;26(4):396–402.

77. Boller M, Kellett-Gregory L, Shofer FS, et al. The clinical practice of CPCR in small animals: an internet-based survey. J Vet Emerg Crit Care 2010;20(6): 558–70.

78. Cole SG, Otto CM, Hughes D. Cardiopulmonary cerebral resus- citation in small animals – a clinical practice review. Part II. J Vet Emerg Crit Care 2003;13(1): 13–23.

Update on the Management of Neonatal Sepsis in Horses

Jon Palmer, VMD

KEYWORDS

- Severe sepsis • Septic shock • Fluid therapy • Antimicrobials • Vasoactive agents
- Antimediator therapy • Glucose control • Corticosteroids

KEY POINTS

- The diagnosis of sepsis, severe sepsis, and septic shock is based on clinical judgment. None of the associated clinical signs or immediately available laboratory findings are specific for sepsis, so management must be initiated before a definitive diagnosis is reached.
- As important as selecting the most appropriate antimicrobial is, both early initiation of treatment and insuring the dose and frequency will allow adequate drug levels in the face of sepsis and shock, which will change many aspects of the antimicrobial's pharmacodynamics.
- Plasma therapy may not only deliver useful immunoglobulins and other immunologically important factors but can also serve other important functions, such as aiding in the repair of the damaged endothelial glycocalyx layer, which is vital in preserving fluid balance and volemia in the neonate.
- Fluid therapy should follow the "Goldilocks approach." Too much fluid is dangerous. Too little fluid is dangerous. A balance is needed.
- Although many approaches have been tried, no antimediator therapy has been successful in mitigating the damage caused by uncontrolled sepsis and, in fact, many therapies which are based on experimental models would seem be rational have actually increased mortality in clinical trials in man.

INTRODUCTION

Development of a bacterial infection is a common cause of morbidity and mortality in neonatal foals. It is not only the most common cause of fatality during this period but also the most important comorbidity of other neonatal diseases, such as prematurity and neonatal encephalopathy, increasing the risk of a more complicated course and a fatal outcome. The concept of sepsis is ancient, being described by both the Egyptians and Hippocrates,[1,2] but it was Schottmueller[3] in 1914 who first established a

Graham French Neonatal Section, Connelly Intensive Care Unit, New Bolton Center, University of Pennsylvania, 382 West Street Road, Kennett Square, PA 19348, USA
E-mail address: jepalmer@vet.upenn.edu

Vet Clin Equine 30 (2014) 317–336
http://dx.doi.org/10.1016/j.cveq.2014.04.005
0749-0739/14/$ – see front matter © 2014 Elsevier Inc. All rights reserved.

link between the presence of pathogenic microbes in the bloodstream and the development of systemic symptoms and signs. In Schottmueller's words, "Septicemia is a state of microbial invasion from a portal of entry into the blood stream which causes signs of illness." Sepsis, the host's response to infection, is a continuum of clinical syndromes ranging from signs, such as fever and catabolism secondary to a localized, well-controlled infection, to septic shock with its refractory shock and its accompanying multiorgan dysfunction. Sepsis results from the dysregulation of the systemic host response to cascading inflammatory and anti-inflammatory mediators induced by infecting organisms.[4]

During the last 2 decades, as the complexities of the sepsis response have begun to be understood, many ideas have emerged aimed at managing clinical sepsis by mitigating the damage caused by the inflammatory response while simultaneously preserving the ability to purge the initiating microbial invaders as well as resist secondary infections. Working from bench to patient side, many initially promising therapies have often fallen flat, which is a reflection of the complexity of the response with multiple redundant pathways making control of the cascading responses problematic. The evidence of efficacy in the treatment of sepsis comes from large blinded clinical studies in adult humans. There is some evidence from human neonatal studies, but unfortunately, there are no adequately powered clinical studies in septic neonatal foals to lend evidence to any of the approaches to therapy. Therefore, at best, evidence has been "borrowed" from human trials to direct many of the clinical approaches to septic neonatal foals. This approach is dangerous because the host response may differ greatly.

There is some information from sepsis models in foals and horses, but we need to heed the lesions from human medicine that many of the most promising approaches to managing sepsis based on models have actually resulted in increased fatality rates when used in clinical settings.[4,5] Another important lesson to learn from human medicine is the reliance on models that use endotoxin to induce sepsis may result in misplaced confidence in the usefulness of the therapy in clinical situations.[5] Although endotoxin models may help in understanding many aspects of sepsis, more clinically relevant models that involve multiple initiators of sepsis are more likely to yield more valuable therapeutic information.[2,5] The movement to more clinically realistic models of sepsis would be a big step forward in the development of effective management approaches to equine sepsis. Until then, the most reliable methods to manage sepsis in the neonatal foal will remain grounded on the same cornerstones that were established more than 2 decades ago: infection control (antimicrobials, plasma, drainage when possible), cardiovascular support (fluids, inopressors), respiratory support (intranasal oxygen insufflation/ventilation), and nutritional support.[6]

THE SEPTIC NEONATAL FOAL

Many terms have been used to define "sepsis" since Schottmueller first established a link between the clinical signs and infection.[3] The often interchangeable use of terms, such as infection, septicemia, bacteremia, and sepsis syndrome, has led to some confusion. However, using the concept of sepsis as the host response to infection and a hierarchy of terms based on severity, the associated terminology becomes relatively simple (**Box 1**).[4] In 1991, Bone and colleagues[7] coined the concept of systemic inflammatory response syndrome. It is a useful term when describing the pathogens of sepsis but their original definition, based on patient temperature, heart rate, respiratory rate or P_{CO_2}, and white blood cell count, was designed to cast a broad net to include as many patients as possible in early sepsis therapeutic trials with the knowledge that the nonspecific nature of the inclusion criteria would mean enrolling many

---

Box 1
Definitions

Infection: a pathologic process caused by the invasion of normally sterile tissue or fluid or body cavity by pathogenic or potentially pathogenic microorganisms.

Sepsis: the clinical syndrome defined by the presence of both infection and a systemic inflammatory response.

Severe sepsis: sepsis complicated by organ dysfunction, usually acute circulatory failure characterized by hypoperfusion unexplained by other causes and readily corrected by volume resuscitation alone.

Septic shock: severe sepsis plus acute circulatory failure characterized by persistent hypoperfusion unexplained by other causes and despite adequate volume resuscitation.

Data from Vincent JL. Clinical sepsis and septic shock—definition, diagnosis and management principles. Langenbecks Arch Surg 2008;393:817–24; and Bone RC, Balk RA, Cerra FB, et al. Definition for sepsis and organ failure and guidelines for the use of innovative therapies in sepsis. Chest 1992;101:1644–55.

---

patients that did not actually suffer from sepsis. Although more recently the definition has been expanded to a longer list of possible signs as well as the results of blood assays of inflammatory mediators, some have considered the term outdated because understanding of the pathophysiology of sepsis has increased.[4] It is of little use in the identification of clinical sepsis in neonatal foals.

In 1988, Brewer and Koterba[8,9] proposed a foal sepsis score to identify sepsis in hospitalized neonatal foals. Their scoring system has been widely embraced and is a valuable epidemiologic tool, but, as acknowledged in the original paper, has some shortcomings when applied to individual cases. The accuracy and reproducibility of fibrinogen and immunoglobulin G (IgG) levels used in the scheme depend on the technique used. The band count and identification of toxic changes in neutrophils also used in the score are laboratory-dependent. The population used to develop the score had a high incidence of prematurity and placentitis, rendering it less useful for postnatal infections and mature foals. It is unfortunate in the 25 years since the scoring scheme was proposed that it has not been proven in a large independent population, a process necessary to validate any risk scoring scheme.[10] In the original population, there were several foals with false negative scores and, in a small population reported by Peek and colleagues,[11] the scoring scheme had a sensitivity of 74% in predicting bacteremia. The occurrence of these false negative test results, which have also been anecdotally noted in the author's neonatal population, is important in light of the importance of initiating early antimicrobial therapy (see later discussion). As noted by Brewer and Koterba[8,9] the sepsis score was developed as an aid to diagnosis but was not intended to be used to direct decisions on the institution of antimicrobial therapy. Some of the false negative cases may be because the examination is performed too early in the clinical course for the expected changes (such as with the delay in increase in fibrinogen) and in others the scoring system may fail because the case comes from a population different from that which produced the scoring system. In the author's experience, use of the score on an individual case may dangerously delay initiation of antimicrobials.

Diagnosing sepsis can be difficult. Blood cultures are useful, but cases are not consistently bacteremic, and rapid identification of blood pathogens is not widely available. None of the clinical signs or common laboratory findings is specific for sepsis. The occurrence of multiple, complex underlying disease processes often confuses the clinical picture. The ideal marker of infection, which should be sensitive enough to detect the presence of infection in patients with minimal or even no host response, specific enough to discriminate infection from other stimuli that may induce a systemic inflammatory response, should be present early in the course of the disease, should be rapidly and conveniently measured, and should be of prognostic significance, is yet to be identified. Diagnosis must thus rely on a strong clinical suspicion supported by the combined presence of several of the signs of sepsis (**Boxes 2 and 3**).

Box 2
Some indications of sepsis in the neonatal foal

Clinical signs
- Fever/hypothermia
- Tachycardia/inappropriate bradycardia
- Tachypnea
- Hypoperfusion
  - Poor pulse quality/poor arterial fill/poor arterial tone
  - Arterial hypotension (low blood pressure)
  - Cold legs/hooves
  - Increased venous capacitance
  - Decreased urine output
- Edema (especially asymmetric edema)
- Oral small vessel injection
- Coronitis
- Nasal/facial erythema/altered skin perfusion
- Oral/aural petechia

Generalized hematological/inflammatory reaction
- Leukopenia/neutropenia (sometimes neutrophilia)
- Decreased urine output (not associated with hypoperfusion)
- Unexplained lactatemia/increased base deficit

Signs of organ dysfunction
- Hypoxemia despite intranasal oxygen insufflation (suspect acute lung injury)
- Depression/somnolence (in the absence of neonatal encephalopathy)
- Unexplained alteration in renal function
  - Rising creatinine/slow decrease in birth creatinine levels
  - Low urine output
  - Isosthenuric urine
  - Abnormal urinalysis
- Hypoglycemia/hyperglycemia
- Thrombocytopenia/disseminated intravascular coagulation
- Unexplained alteration in liver function tests (hyperbilirubinemia)
- Intolerance to feeding (gastrointestinal dysmotility)

> **Box 3**
> **Organ dysfunction common in sepsis**
>
> - Cardiovascular
>   - Hypotension
>   - Tachycardia/arrhythmias
>   - Lactatemia (secondary to hypoperfusion)
>   - Cardiac failure
> - Respiratory
>   - Tachypnea/respiratory distress
>   - Hypoxia/hypercapnia
>   - Acute respiratory distress syndrome
> - Kidneys—acute kidney injury
>   - Increasing plasma creatinine/slow decrease in birth creatinine levels
>   - Decreasing urine output
>   - Fluid overload
>   - Electrolyte imbalances
> - Central nervous system—nonfocal septic encephalopathy
>   - Depression
>   - Weakness
>   - Somnolence
> - Metabolic
>   - Lactatemia (not from anaerobic metabolism)
>   - Loss of glycemic control/hypoglycemia/hyperglycemia
> - Coagulopathies
>   - Thrombocytopenia
>   - Disseminated intravascular coagulation
> - Altered adrenal function
>   - Adrenal exhaustion
>   - Loss of receptor sensitivity
> - Gastrointestinal
>   - Ileus/distention/reflux/dysmotility
>   - Diarrhea
>
> *Data from* Angus DC, van der Poll T. Severe sepsis and septic shock. N Engl J Med 2013;369(9):840–51.

The final arbitrator is clinical judgment based on experience, keeping in mind the importance of early intervention.

MANAGEMENT STRATEGIES IN NEONATAL SEPSIS

This discussion focuses on the management of severe sepsis and septic shock because these are the most challenging, and despite the increase in understanding, continue to have poor outcomes. There has been an increasing realization of the importance of early resuscitation on positive outcomes from severe sepsis and septic shock in man.[12–14] The same is undoubtedly true for the neonatal foal. Management of foals with severe sepsis essentially comprises 4 key aspects: infection control, hemodynamic support, immunomodulatory interventions, and metabolic/endocrine support.

Infection Control

Control of infection relies on appropriate antimicrobial therapy, plasma therapy, and identification of any infected focus with local treatment when possible. Searches for an infected focus through complete physical examinations and imaging should be made repeatedly. The "big six" locations of sepsis should be kept in mind when trying to identify a source, with the search initially focusing on the umbilical remnants, lungs, gastrointestinal tract, urinary tract, physes/joints, and catheters. Identification of the focus may allow culturing of infected material, directed local therapy (eg, joint flush, physis curettage, removal of catheter), and also may help direct antimicrobial therapy based on typical pathogens found in the area when culture results are not yet available.

Antimicrobials

Appropriate antimicrobial therapy should be begun within an hour of development of hypoperfusion in cases with severe sepsis or septic shock.[14–17] Initial antimicrobial choice is empiric. The author focuses the choice by keeping track of both community-acquired isolates' and nosocomial isolates' sensitivities over the past 3 years and bases his antimicrobial choice on this information, along with any patient-specific clues that may be helpful, such as infection location and recent farm history. In approximately 60% of cases of neonatal foal sepsis, no organisms will be isolated. Once started, antimicrobial drugs should be continued for 7 to 10 days with longer courses considered in patients who have a slow clinical response or immunologic deficiencies, including persistent neutropenia. Biomarkers of infection, such as hyperfibrinogenemia, may be used to determine the need for continued antibiotic therapy.[4] Achieving optimal target levels rapidly is as important as early initiation of appropriate antimicrobials.[6] Pharmacokinetics are affected by changes that occur during sepsis, so information from drug behavior in normal individuals is of limited value when treating septic foals.[18–20] However, there are few studies testing drug levels in septic foals. It should also be recalled that there is no one correct antimicrobial dose because the level achieved will vary depending on many host factors and the level required will vary depending on pathogen characteristics. Therefore, there is no one dose that is appropriate for all situations (**Table 1**).

Plasma therapy

Plasma therapy may also be helpful, although currently there is no evidence to support this notion. Although measuring the IgG may be useful to document low levels because of failure of passive transfer or secondary to sepsis-mediated catabolism, it should not be the deciding factor for giving a plasma transfusion. Despite having a large quantity of IgG acquired from passive transfer, useful antibodies may not be present. The IgG present did not prevent sepsis, but antibodies in the transfused hyperimmune plasma might be helpful. Other factors in plasma may also be helpful. It should be noted that high levels of IgG can be immunosuppressive,[21] but in sepsis with its associated catabolism, these levels are rarely reached even with repeated plasma transfusions.

Table 1
Suggested dosing of selected antimicrobials for septic foals

Antimicrobial	Dosage	Frequency	Route	Notes
Ceftiofur sodium	10 mg/kg	QID	IV	With high doses, should be infused slowly over at least 20 min
	1.6 mg/kg/h	CRI	IV	Begin CRI after a bolus dose
Ticarcillin/clavulanic acid	50–100 mg/kg	QID	IV	
	8.3–16 mg/kg/h	CRI	IV	Begin CRI after a bolus dose
K Penicillin	20,000–50,000 U/kg	QID	IV	In severe cases, may be given every 3–4 h
	8,000 U/kg/h	CRI	IV	Begin CRI after a bolus dose
Cefuroxime Na	50–100 mg/kg/d	IV	Divided TID, QID	Doses up to 200 mg/kg/d used in severe infections
Cefuroxime axetil	30 mg/kg/d	PO	Divided BID, TID	
Gentamicin	16–20 mg/kg	SID	IV	Ideally drug levels should be measured and dose adjusted with the goal of peak (30 min) >40 μg/mL and trough (23 h) <2 μg/mL
Amikacin	30–35 mg/kg	SID	IV	Ideally drug levels should be measured and dose adjusted with goal peak (30 min) >60 μg/mL and trough (23 h) <2 μg/mL
Trimethoprim potentiated sulfa	30 mg/kg	BID	PO, IV	
Doxycycline	10 mg/kg	BID	PO	
Minocycline	4 mg/kg	BID	PO	

In general, the use of plasma transfusions, which should act to enhance the immune response to sepsis, may be more rational than the use of anti-inflammatory drugs in light of the down-regulation of many immune responses. Although the innate immune system is often generally activated in sepsis, the adaptive immune system is more often in a state of marked immune suppression. This phase of sepsis-induced immune dysregulation occurs early and may be the dominating immunologic feature in a substantial proportion of septic patients. If this is the case, it makes little sense to administer potent anti-inflammatory agents to treat septic patients when immune reconstitution in the form of plasma therapy might be needed instead.[21,22]

Sepsis and fluid therapy are known to decrease the endothelial glycocalyx layer. Destruction of the endothelial glycocalyx layer is associated with a proinflammatory response, platelet adhesion and microthrombosis, and development of a leaky vasculature. There is evidence that albumin from plasma therapy may help restore the glycocalyx layer, protecting against these problems[23] and is an example of one of the many positive effects plasma transfusion may have beyond immunoglobulin transfer when used in septic foals.

Hemodynamic Support

Fluid therapy

Authorities agree that the most important facet concerning hemodynamic resuscitation is rapid initiation.[12] However, most other aspects of fluid therapy, such as type of fluid and how aggressively fluid therapy should be pursued, have come under scrutiny over the past few years. The 25-year-old promise that 20 mL of colloids would be equal to 100 mL of crystalloids and colloids would mobilize intestinal fluids, drawing them into the vasculature, has gone unfulfilled.[24] One reason is that the assumptions Ernest Starling theorized in 1896 do not fully explain the behavior of fluids during sepsis[24] and simply are not true in septic shock. Major revisions of Starling's theories take into account the importance of the endothelial glycocalyx layer in producing the colloid oncotic pressure and determining transcapillary flow.[25] These new theories explain observations of fluid shifts in sepsis and the discovery that colloid osmotic pressure (COP) properties of plasma or plasma substitutes add little or nothing to plasma volume resuscitation because plasma and interstitial COP are similar when the glycocalyx is stripped, resulting in little transcapillary flow.[26] In addition, transendothelial hydrostatic pressure difference is low in cases of shock, also resulting in limited transcapillary flow.[24] This theory explains the observation in blind clinical trials that the ratio of colloids to crystalloids needed to achieve clinical resuscitation is near 1:1.3 and not the 1:5 originally theorized.[25] Therefore, the volume of crystalloids and colloids retained intravascularly is very similar in septic shock. Perhaps some of the success of colloids seen in early colloid versus crystalloid studies when the volume given was adjusted to be "fair" to the crystalloid side (eg, much higher volumes of crystalloids were given than colloids) really reflect the negative effects of high volumes rather than the positive effects of colloids. It has become evident in man from at least 6 well-designed blinded prospective clinical trials that synthetic colloids have no resuscitation advantage over crystalloids and at the same time the colloids are significantly associated with other comorbidities (renal failure, coagulopathy, liver dysfunction) and higher late-term mortality.[25] The use of synthetic colloids cannot be justified in neonatal foals until evidence from large prospective clinical trials is performed.

It should also be noted that the chloride concentration of the chosen crystalloid is important. The acute hyperchloremia induced by high-chloride fluid therapy can adversely affect urine output via feedback mechanisms on the macula densa. Giving more saline in an attempt to increase urine output can result in a vicious cycle. Fluid therapy–induced hyperchloremia has been associated with acute kidney injury and may be a proinflammatory stimulus.[27]

Aggressive fluid resuscitation, which has been a mainstay of management of septic shock,[28,29] has been recently questioned and critiqued as being weakly supported by evidence.[30] Indeed, cohort studies in man have reported an association between positive fluid balance and mortality.[31–35] Recently, The Fluid Expansion as Supportive Therapy (FEAST) study compared fluid boluses of 20 to 40 mL/kg with no bolus in more than 3000 acutely ill African children.[36] FEAST reported a significantly increased mortality risk in the group randomized to the fluid bolus arm. Fluid overload and aggressive volume resuscitation are certainly related. Rapid infusion of fluids in normal individuals increasing vascular volume may disrupt the endothelial glycocalyx layer, resulting in capillary leak in the absence of any other abnormality.[24] Thus, the results of the FEAST study could reflect the inclusion of a large number of participants for whom fluid administration may indeed be intrinsically deleterious, rather than leading to the conclusion that fluid administration is intrinsically deleterious in septic shock.[36]

Although fluid resuscitation should be performed using boluses as opposed to continuous infusion as previously suggested[37] and fluids alone are sometimes sufficient to restore hemodynamic stability, overzealous fluid administration should be avoided. The clinical principle is to give enough early on to achieve survivable perfusion and not normal perfusion and then to follow with judicious fluid volumes. Sepsis is often a problem of vascular capacitance as opposed to true hypovolemia. Restoring vascular tone (venous and arterial) with vasopressors as well as fluid resuscitation in a balanced approach may be better than relying on fluids alone. It has even been suggested that not only should the peripheral circulation be allowed to shut down but in fact it should be encouraged to do so. In this view, central circulation perfusing vital organs should be maintained, but infusing large volumes of fluids in an attempt to fill the vascular tree as clinically indicated by warm legs and good peripheral pulse pressure will result in increased vascular leak and fluid overload and its associated adverse effects. The important clinical question that needs to be addressed is not should patients with septic shock receive fluid resuscitation, but rather, how much fluid resuscitation is most optimal.[38] Currently the author suggests using the "Goldilocks approach." Too much fluid is dangerous. Too little fluid is dangerous. A balance is needed by initially fluid loading (through 20 mL/kg boluses) and then adding inopressor therapy when possible or relying on endogenous inopressor support when not, because fluid volumes are slowed to a maintenance level or less. We should not try to return normal perfusion with aggressive unrestrained fluid therapy alone. In any case, the foal's need for additional fluids should be assessed on an ongoing basis. The problem is that there is no clinical indicator or indeed expensive monitoring modality that will tell us when we have reached the balance. We can only rely on our imperfect clinical judgment.

Vasoactive agents

Vasoactive agents are often needed to maintain adequate perfusion in patients with septic shock and they are frequently started early, even before fluid therapy goals have been met. Vasoactive agents should only be used when intensive care with continuous rate infusion using intravenous infusion pumps and continuous monitoring is possible. The most commonly used drugs for hemodynamic support include dobutamine, dopamine, norepinephrine, epinephrine, and vasopressin. As there is no consistent evidence for or against individual drugs, current choices largely come down to personal preference based on anecdotal experience. The author's current first choice is the combination of dobutamine and vasopressin, but when using these agents, it should always be remembered that because of a large number of variables, it is difficult to predict the individual's response to the different agents (**Table 2**). If one agent or combination of agents seems ineffective, then others should be tried. Use of these agents should be accompanied by frequent reassessment of their need and the foal's response. With the possible exception of vasopressin, the maximum effect of an infused dose should be seen within 10 to 15 minutes. Therefore, the dose of these agents should be reassessed and adjusted several times an hour until the lowest effective dose is found. As the foal's clinical condition changes, the doses should also be reassessed because the effect of these agents will vary significantly with the foal's condition (acidosis/alkalosis, fluid status, liver/renal function, inflammatory mediators). Which endpoints should be targeted for vasoactive therapy remain unclear. Normalization of global hemodynamic parameters does not necessarily indicate that tissue perfusion and oxygenation are adequate. On the contrary, increasing

Table 2
Suggested doses of vasoactive drugs in the neonatal foal

Drug	Initial Dose	Usual Dose Range	Maximum Dose	Comments
Dobutamine	5 μg/kg/min	3–20 μg/kg/min	40 μg/kg/min	At low doses, primarily inotrope; at higher doses, inopressor
Dopamine	5 μg/kg/min	3–20 μg/kg/min	20 μg/kg/min	Often combined with dobutamine
Norepinephrine	0.4 μg/kg/min	0.2–2 μg/kg/min	3 μg/kg/min	Primarily thought of as a pressor but also has inotropic properties; often combined with dobutamine
Epinephrine	0.4 μg/kg/min	0.2–2 μg/kg/min	3 μg/kg/min	Primarily thought of as an inotrope but also has pressor properties; often combined with norepinephrine
Vasopressin	0.5 mU/kg/min	0.25–2 mU/kg/min	2 mU/kg/min	Has many complex actions but primarily a pressor; often combined with dobutamine

blood pressure to what is considered normal may decrease perfusion and oxygen to some tissues. An important example is a decrease in gastrointestinal blood flow. Diminution of gut barrier function has been suggested as a mechanism for the development of secondary infections and multiple organ failure in patients with septic shock.[6] Nevertheless, until a better means of measuring and monitoring tissue oxygenation is found, ongoing vasoactive therapy must be based on clinical response and global hemodynamic and oxygenation parameters, including mixed venous oxygen saturation and blood lactate levels. Caution should be used when following lactate levels because there are many aspects of sepsis that will stimulate lactate production unrelated to oxygen delivery. The objective is to monitor for a decrease in lactate levels as a positive indication of improved perfusion but not to expect a return to normal levels. A complete discussion of the use of vasoactive agents is beyond the scope of this review.

Respiratory support
Although supporting hemodynamics will help optimize oxygen delivery to tissues, optimizing pulmonary transfer of oxygen is also important. There are many changes that occur in septic shock that interfere with oxygen uptake in the lungs, including the development of pulmonary hypertension with associated right-to-left shunting in the neonate and significant mismatching secondary to abnormal vascular control in the lungs. Another consideration is that 25% of oxygen consumption during septic shock in a patient in respiratory distress may be used to support respiration. If the work of breathing can be minimized and the matching of ventilation to perfusion can be optimized, then the neonate has a better chance of overcoming septic shock and not suffering from a lack of oxygen delivery. All neonates suffering from septic

shock are usually placed on intranasal oxygen to decrease the work of breathing and optimize gas transport. Early in the course of the disease, consideration should be given to ventilation, which will further decrease the work of breathing, increase cardiovascular function, and make early respiratory failure easier to manage, and early ventilation may improve outcome. When ventilated, a modest positive end expiratory pressure (PEEP) should be used to decrease the work of breathing and airway resistance and decrease hypoxia and the need for high F_{IO2} levels in attempts to avoid hyperoxia. Inhaled nitric oxide may be useful in reversing the pulmonary hypertension that is secondary to septic shock. Recently, there has been evidence that, although oxygen therapy may be important, titrating oxygen therapy to achieve normal oxygen levels instead of hyperoxia may be important in limiting negative effects of oxygen therapy.[39]

Antimediator Therapy

Infection triggers a complex host response in which both proinflammatory and antiinflammatory mechanisms participate to clear infection and promote tissue recovery, but can also cause organ injury and allow secondary infections.[2] Proinflammatory reactions, which are directed at eliminating invading pathogens, may simultaneously result in collateral tissue damage, whereas anti-inflammatory responses, which attempt to limit local and systemic tissue damage, can result in enhanced susceptibility to secondary infections.[2] The underlying rationale for antimediator-based sepsis therapies is simple. Infection by diverse pathogens stimulates pathogen-associated molecular pattern receptors, resulting in common pathway responses characterized by the excessive systemic release of host-derived, humoral factors leading to multiple organ failure, vascular collapse, and death. Interventions that could block these common pathways could potentially act therapeutically against a wide array of pathogens that cause sepsis. This hypothesis has proven problematic because it has become evident that the same mediators that cause general inflammation and harm in sepsis, such as cytokines, complement components, and coagulation activators, also have protective roles in defending the host by purging the pathogen and preventing secondary microbial invasion. In addition, many of the most important parts of these complicated schemes have numerous, highly redundant activation pathways and networks. Blocking one signaling pathway is not sufficient to terminate acute inflammatory processes, as others will be activated and compensate for the inhibited pathway. In addition, pattern recognition receptors are not just distinguishing "self" from "nonself" molecules. Identical receptors also recognize danger signals, "alarmins," originating from damaged host tissues. Therefore, targeting such signaling and response pathways has the potential to be of no therapeutic value or perhaps even to be harmful as demonstrated in several therapeutic trials in man.[2,22] In man, more than 40 approaches to target signaling and response pathways, which showed great promise in clinical models, either failed to show benefit in human therapeutic trials or were found to be harmful (**Box 4**).

Although there have been no large prospective studies examining antimediator therapy in foals, there are a few that have traditionally been used, including, among others, flunixin meglumine, Polymyxin B, pentoxifylline, and antiendotoxin antibodies. Flunixin has one of the longest traditions because it was discovered to help offset deleterious hemodynamic effects of endotoxin in acute experimental disease models in the 1980s and more recently to have antimediator effects against matrix metalloproteinases.[40–46] It is commonly used on the clinic floor.[47] Unfortunately, there are no prospective clinical trials to confirm that it is indeed useful in the treatment of clinical sepsis. The author has anecdotally noticed consistent renal dysfunction when it is used in septic

Box 4
Selected antimediator approaches that have failed to reproducibly benefit septic human patients

High-dose steroids

IV immunoglobulin

Antiendotoxin antibodies (*E coli* J5)

Heparin

Polymyxin B conjugants

Polymyxin B columns

Bactericidal permeability increasing protein

Antithrombin

Tight glycemic control

Stress dose steroids

Albumin hemoperfusion

TNF mAb

Chimeric TNF mAb

Humanized TNF mAb

TNF-antigen binding fragment of immunoglobulin

sTNFR1:Fc

sTNFR2:Fc

Antilipid A E5 mAb

Antilipid A HA1A mAb

Complement component 1 esterase inhibitor

Tissue factor pathway inhibitor

Recombinant human activated protein C

Nematode anticoagulant protein c2

Recombinant high-density lipoprotein and phospholipid complexes

Eritoran tetrasodium

Anti-CD14 mAb

Interleukin-1 receptor antagonist

PAF receptor antagonists

PAF-acetyl hydrolase

Ibuprofen

Anti-β2 integrin

Nitric oxide synthase inhibitors

Growth hormone

Bradykinin inhibitors

TAK (Takeda) 242

Lactoferrin

Abbreviations: Fc, crystallizable fraction of immunoglobulin; mAb, monoclonal antibody; PAF, platelet-activating factor; sTNFR, soluble tumor necrosis factor receptor; TNF, tumor necrosis factor.

Data from Artenstein AW, Higgins TL, Opal SM. Sepsis and scientific revolutions. Crit Care Med 2013;41:2770–2.

neonates, especially if there were indications of pre-existing renal compromise. As there is no good evidence of its usefulness and there is a possible renal risk, the author does not use flunixin in septic neonates.

Polymyxin B has shown some encouraging evidence in experimental endotoxemia models in horses with improvement of clinical signs (reduced fever and tachycardia) and decreased mediator levels.[48–50] Because of the significant risk of renal damage, in man, Polymyxin B is bound to a filter in a hemoadsorption technique (continuous renal replacement therapy). Currently, trials in man have not resolved the usefulness of Polymyxin B in septic patients.[51] One reason for this may be that Polymyxin B does not bind endotoxin from all gram-negative bacteria equally.[52] Because of the risk of renal disease when administered intravenously and the lack of evidence from clinical trials, the author does not currently use this treatment in septic neonates.

Similar to flunixin and Polymyxin B, pentoxifylline has shown antimediator activity in experimental sepsis in horses against matrix metalloproteinases[45] and has been shown to help offset deleterious hemodynamic effects of endotoxin in experimental sepsis in horses.[40] Small clinical trials have shown promise of a positive effect in human neonatal sepsis.[53,54] However, with no clinical trial evidence and no reasonably priced parenteral formulation, it has not become part of the author's treatment regime for neonatal foal sepsis.

Whether the presence of antiendotoxin antibody (induced by immunization with J5 Escherichia coli or a re-mutant of Salmonella typhimurium) is beneficial in sepsis is not clear. Based on their findings studying an experimental model of endotoxemia in the horse, Durando and colleagues[49] concluded that antiendotoxin antibody had no positive effects on endotoxemia and, under certain conditions, may exacerbate the actions of endotoxin. In clinical trials in man, there has also been a lack of success.[55–58] Others have found encouraging results in small studies of foals[11] or adult horses[59] receiving hyperimmune plasma rich in antiendotoxin antibodies.

SUPPORTIVE THERAPY

General supportive therapy can be very important in achieving a positive outcome in neonatal sepsis. Because of the catabolism of sepsis, loss of glucose control that often accompanies sepsis and the negative effects poor nutrition has on the immune system, nutritional support is both essential and problematic. Foals with severe sepsis or septic shock should not receive enteral feeding until they are fully resuscitated. Regardless of their blood glucose level, they can benefit from glucose infusions. They should be begun on an infusion rate of 4 mg/kg/min of glucose and gradually increase to 8 mg/kg/min as long as they do not become hyperglycemic. This latter rate of glucose infusion will deliver an energy level of approximately 40 kcal/kg/d. If the foal becomes hyperglycemic, a continuous rate infusion (CRI) of regular insulin can be effective. Because neonatal foals, even when septic, are rarely insulin resistant, the infusion should be begun at a very small dose (initially 0.0025 U/kg/h), doubling the infusion rate every 4 hours until the glucose level is controlled or the infusion rate is greater than 0.2 U/kg/h. Special care needs to be followed when infusing insulin, such as preconditioning the infusion lines, special handling of the insulin, and frequently following blood glucose levels to avoid both hypoglycemia and further hyperglycemia. Once there is moderation of the hyperglycemia, the glucose infusion rate should be increased to the goal of 8 mg/kg/min. When the initial problem is severe hypoglycemia secondary to sepsis glucose infusion, rates may need to be increased to 20 mg/kg/min or more to correct the problem. When delivering glucose-containing fluids, it is important to calculate the infusion rate carefully in milligrams per kilogram per minute, instead of milliliter per hour of a glucose-containing fluid or just adding dextrose to the infused fluids to avoid serious iatrogenic errors. If the neonatal foal suffering from severe sepsis or septic shock is tolerating an 8 mg/kg/min glucose infusion and receiving plasma transfusions that will provide albumin and other proteins, further nutritional support such as parenteral nutrition with the addition of lipids and amino acids can be deferred until the foal is fully resuscitated.

Tight Glucose Control

For the past decade, beginning with the study by Van den Berghe[60] in 2001, the use of tight glucose control in sepsis has been controversial in man. Many studies in septic adult humans have shown that the duration and intensity of hyperglycemia are directly related to outcomes.[61] Hollis and coworkers[62] showed that both hypoglycemia and hyperglycemia were associated with poor outcomes in neonatal foals, although that study did not take into account the normal physiologic changes in glucose blood levels during the first 24 hours in foals so that the effect of hypoglycemia may have only reflected the foal's age at admission. High glucose levels may affect several aspects of physiology that are thought to play a role in outcomes. Its effects include oxidative injury, inducing a proinflammatory response, producing clotting abnormalities, causing vascular reactivity, and decreasing immune system effectiveness. Hyperglycemia may compromise all major components of the innate immune system, including phagocytosis and opsonization, glycosylation, and inactivation of circulating immunoglobulins. These effects may contribute to an increased risk of infection. Preventing hyperglycemia with insulin could protect organs from glucose-related damage, especially in the kidney, where it is thought that hyperglycemia may induce renal mesangial cell apoptosis and increase the risk of acute kidney injury and renal failure. However, it is not known whether glucose results in pathologic abnormality or is a marker of the pathologic abnormality. Initial studies in man suggested that the glucose be tightly controlled with a target level of 80 to 108 mg/dL, but scrutiny of the initial results suggested that attempting to achieve this tight control put patients at risk of hypoglycemia and increased risk of death.[61] In the most definitive study to date, the Normoglycemia in Intensive Care Evaluation-Survival Using Glucose Algorithm Regulation (NICE-SUGAR) trial[63] suggested that a blood glucose target of 180 mg/dL or less resulted in lower mortality than did a target of 80 to 108 mg/dL in man. Based on this information, until clinical trials are performed on neonatal foals, it would be reasonable to attempt to keep glucose levels less than 180 mg/dL and/or prevent significant spilling of glucose in the urine.

Corticosteroid Replacement Therapy

The role of adrenal insufficiency and the use of corticosteroids as potential adjunctive therapy in sepsis have been proposed for decades. Initial efforts, centered around the concept of sepsis as an excessive and dysregulated proinflammatory response, primarily studied short courses of high-dose corticosteroids intended for inflammatory suppression. This approach failed. More recently, a condition called critical illness–related corticosteroid insufficiency (CIRCI) has been used to describe a group of critically ill patients who seemingly have an inadequate cortisol response relative to their degree of illness. A similar group with CIRCI has been described in hospitalized foals,[64–68] although at least one study of septic hospitalized foals showed conflicting results.[69]

Although it is still unclear if the CIRCI is a marker of the severity of the disease or if it plays a role in the pathogenesis, its recognition has renewed interest in the use of corticosteroid therapy in sepsis with the aim of hormone replacement therapy instead of the use of pharmacologic doses. A study of critically ill children showed that relative adrenal insufficiency was associated with a greater need for the number of catecholamines, a greater duration of catecholamine requirement, and a greater need for volume resuscitation.[70] This study supported the concept that relative adrenal

---

Box 5
Steps in the management of the neonatal foal with severe sepsis or septic shock

- Take blood cultures and cultures of other sites before antibiotic administration
- Administer broad-spectrum antibiotics as soon as possible
  - Consider adding first dose to initial fluid bolus
  - Insure adequate dose and interval for septic shock
  - Consider CRI for β-lactams
- Fluid bolus challenge therapy to predefined clinical goals
  - 10–20 mL/kg boluses
  - Reassess if goal is met between each bolus
- Begin respiratory support/monitor arterial blood gases
  - Intranasal oxygen insufflation
  - Ventilation in select cases
  - Stand and turn at least every 2 hours
  - Positional support (keeping sternal) in select cases
- Plasma therapy
  - At least 1–2 L
  - Can be given as part of fluid bolus challenge (insure compatibility first)
  - Can be used as maintenance fluid
- Begin glucose therapy
  - 4 mg/kg/min increasing to 8 mg/kg/min
  - Watch and manage blood glucose levels
- Measure serum lactate concentrations
  - Take baseline sample
  - Monitor for changes
- Administer vasoactive drugs for continued hypoperfusion (may begin before full fluid resuscitation)
  - Dobutamine and vasopressin or
  - Dobutamine and norepinephrine or
  - Epinephrine and norepinephrine
- Consider measuring central venous oxygen saturation; maintain greater than 70%
- Control the source of sepsis as soon as possible
- Consider cortisol replacement therapy
  - Only in cases with septic shock (not responsive to adrenergic therapy)
  - Discontinue once shock resolves
  - Hydrocortisone (50 mg 4 times each day)

insufficiency has functional consequences in pediatric critical illness. With this in mind, recent approaches at corticosteroid therapy have been designed as replacement therapy treating the adrenal insufficiency rather than globally inhibiting the inflammatory response of sepsis. This concept has also been proposed in septic neonatal foals demonstrated to fit the CIRCI classification.[67]

Although there have been no therapeutic trials in foals, there have been several trials in man. An initial positive study using steroid replacement therapy showed benefit in adult patients with septic shock who remained hypotensive after at least 1 hour of resuscitation with fluids and vasopressors (patients with CIRCI whose shock was refractory to adrenergic therapy).[71] They found that only patients who were nonresponders (did not respond to an adrenal stimulation test) benefited from the hydrocortisone therapy. Despite the initial enthusiasm this study generated for the use of cortisol measurements, corticotropin stimulation, and hydrocortisone replacement therapy in both adults and children with septic shock follow-up studies showed conflicting results. The Corticosteroid Therapy for Septic Shock study evaluated the efficacy of hydrocortisone replacement in adult patients with septic shock, based on responder and nonresponder classifications after corticotropin stimulation.[72] This study showed no mortality difference between hydrocortisone-treated patients and placebo-treated patients, irrespective of the responder/nonresponder status. The duration of time until reversal of shock was shorter across all patients treated with hydrocortisone, but there was also a higher rate of shock relapse in the patients treated with hydrocortisone, possibly related to new infections, showing the value of long follow-up in such studies.

Retrospective, pediatric-specific data in man raise some doubts concerning the efficacy of corticosteroids in pediatric septic shock because the use of corticosteroids was found to be an independent predictor of mortality.[73] Therefore, from studies in man, it is apparent that for the pediatric patient with septic shock, the current evidence does not support the use of adjunctive corticosteroids, and some have suggested that the use of corticosteroids may not be benign in these patients.[74] Because of this information, the use of cortisol replacement therapy in septic foals, even those with adrenergic refractory septic shock, cannot be recommended, although some may think it is a justifiable act of desperation in these cases (**Box 5**).

SUMMARY

This article has been a short review of current ideas in the management of sepsis in neonatal foals (see **Box 4**). Therapeutic modulation of sepsis in neonatal foals has been studied in several experimental models. However, an important lesson from human medicine is that even the most promising management techniques proven in experimental models may not only fail on the clinical floor but also increase mortality. Unfortunately, there are no large clinical trials testing the value of therapeutic interventions in neonatal foals. The author's approach to treating septic neonatal foals is largely based on traditions (what has always been done) and beliefs (what is thought should be done based on extrapolation from experimental models) largely because of the lack of foal-specific clinical evidence. Because of this lack of primary evidence, most of this review is based on recent evidence revealed from human clinical studies. The prime medical dictum *Primum Non Nocere* (first, do no harm) should be followed, which has been wrongfully attributed to Hippocrates.[75] To do this, we must be willing to let go of our most cherished traditions and change our most exciting beliefs as new evidence emerges. During the past decade, many of our most basic beliefs in how sepsis and septic shock should be treated have come into question, especially many aspects of fluid therapy. Although it is dangerous to extrapolate from human clinical trials, neither can the results of such trials be ignored. Until results from clinical trials performed on septic neonatal foals emerge, such information forms the basis for the "best guess" on how these very difficult cases should be approached.

REFERENCES

1. Majno G. The ancient riddle of sigma eta psi iota sigma (sepsis). J Infect Dis 1991;163(5):937–45.
2. Angus DC, van der Poll T. Severe sepsis and septic shock. N Engl J Med 2013; 369(9):840–51.
3. Schottmueller H. Wesen und Behandlung der Sepsis. Inn Med 1914;31:257–80.
4. Vincent JL. Clinical sepsis and septic shock—definition, diagnosis and management principles. Langenbecks Arch Surg 2008;393:817–24.
5. Poli-de-Figueiredo LF, Garrido AG, Nakagawa N, et al. Experimental models of sepsis and their clinical relevance. Shock 2008;30(Suppl 1):53–9.
6. Sharma S, Kumar A. Septic shock, multiple organ failure, and acute respiratory distress syndrome. Curr Opin Pulm Med 2003;9:199–209.
7. Bone RC, Balk RA, Cerra FB, et al. Definition for sepsis and organ failure and guidelines for the use of innovative therapies in sepsis. Chest 1992;101:1644–55.
8. Brewer BD, Koterba AM. Development of a scoring system for the early diagnosis of equine neonatal sepsis. Equine Vet J 1988;20(1):18–22.
9. Brewer BD, Koterba AM, Carter L, et al. Comparison of empirically developed sepsis score with a computer generated and weighted scoring system for the identification of sepsis in the equine neonate. Equine Vet J 1988;20(1):23–4.
10. Tacconelli E, Cataldo MA, De Angelis G, et al. Risk scoring and bloodstream infections. Int J Antimicrob Agents 2007;30S:S88–92.
11. Peek SF, Semrad S, McGuirk SM, et al. Prognostic value of clinicopathologic variables obtained at admission and effect of antiendotoxin plasma on survival in septic and critically ill foals. J Vet Intern Med 2006;20(3):569–74.
12. Rivers E, Nguyen B, Havstad S, et al. Early goal-directed therapy in the treatment of severe sepsis and septic shock. N Engl J Med 2001;345:1368–77.
13. Vincent JL, Bernard GR, Beale R, et al. Drotrecogin alfa (activated) treatment in severe sepsis from the global open-label trial ENHANCE. Crit Care Med 2005; 33:2266–77.
14. Kumar A, Roberts D, Wood KE, et al. Duration of hypotension before initiation of effective antimicrobial therapy is the critical determinant of survival in human septic shock. Crit Care Med 2006;34:1589–96.
15. Kumar A, Haery C, Paladugu B, et al. The duration of hypotension before the initiation of antibiotic treatment is a critical determinant of survival in a murine model of Escherichia coli septic shock: association with serum lactate and inflammatory cytokine levels. J Infect Dis 2006;193:251–8.
16. Puskarich MA, Trzeciak S, Shapiro NI, et al. Association between timing of antibiotic administration and mortality from septic shock in patients treated with a quantitative resuscitation protocol. Crit Care Med 2011;39:2066–71.
17. Paul M, Shani V, Muchtar E, et al. Systematic review and meta-analysis of the efficacy of appropriate empiric antibiotic therapy for sepsis. Antimicrob Agents Chemother 2010;54:4851–63.
18. Gálveza R, Luengoa C, Cornejoa R, et al. Higher than recommended amikacin loading doses achieve pharmacokinetic targets without associated toxicity. Int J Antimicrob Agents 2011;38:146–51.

19. Pea F. Plasma pharmacokinetics of antimicrobial agents in critically ill patients. Curr Clin Pharmacol 2013;8(1):5–12.

20. Schwab I, Nimmerjahn F. Intravenous immunoglobulin therapy: how does IgG modulate the immune system? Nat Rev Immunol 2013;13(3):176–89.

21. Hotchkiss RS, Opal S. Immunotherapy for sepsis—A new approach against an ancient foe. N Engl J Med 2010;363:87–9.

22. Artenstein AW, Higgins TL, Opal SM. Sepsis and scientific revolutions. Crit Care Med 2013;41:2770–2.

23. Kozar RA, Peng Z, Zhang R, et al. Plasma restoration of endothelial glycocalyx in a rodent model of hemorrhagic shock. Anesth Analg 2011;112(6):1289–95.

24. Woodcock TE, Woodcock TM. Revised Starling equation and the glycocalyx model of transvascular fluid exchange: an improved paradigm for prescribing intravenous fluid therapy. Br J Anaesth 2012;108(3):384–94.

25. Myburgh JA, Mythen MG. Resuscitation fluids. N Engl J Med 2013;369:1243–51.

26. Jacob M, Bruegger D, Rehm M, et al. The endothelial glycocalyx affords compatibility of Starling's principle and high cardiac interstitial albumin levels. Cardiovasc Res 2007;73(3):575–86.

27. Morgan TJ. The ideal crystalloid – what is 'balanced'? Curr Opin Crit Care 2013; 19(4):299–307.

28. Brierley J, Carcillo JA, Choong K, et al. Clinical practice parameters for hemo-dynamic support of pediatric and neonatal septic shock: 2007 update from the American College of Critical Care Medicine. Crit Care Med 2009;37:666–88.

29. Levy MM, Dellinger RP, Townsend SR, et al. The Surviving Sepsis Campaign: re-sults of an international guideline-based performance improvement program targeting severe sepsis. Crit Care Med 2010;38:367–74.

30. Hilton AK, Bellomo R. A critique of fluid bolus resuscitation in severe sepsis. Crit Care 2012;16:302–7.

31. Vincent JL, Sakr Y, Sprung CL, et al. Sepsis in European intensive care units: results of the SOAP study. Crit Care Med 2006;34:344–53.

32. Boyd JH, Forbes J, Nakada TA, et al. Fluid resuscitation in septic shock: a positive fluid balance and elevated central venous pressure are associated with increased mortality. Crit Care Med 2011;39:259–65.

33. Murphy CV, Schramm GE, Doherty JA, et al. The importance of fluid man-agement in acute lung injury secondary to septic shock. Chest 2009;136: 102–9.

34. Goldstein SL, Somers MJ, Baum MA, et al. Pediatric patients with multi-organ dysfunction syndrome receiving continuous renal replacement therapy. Kidney Int 2005;67:653–8.

35. Maitland K, Kiguli S, Opoka RO, et al. Mortality after fluid bolus in African chil-dren with severe infection. N Engl J Med 2011;364(26):2483–95.

36. Duke T. What the African fluid-bolus trial means. Lancet 2011;378:1685–7.

37. Palmer JE. Fluid therapy in the neonate-not your mother's fluid space. Vet Clin North Am Equine Pract 2004;20(1):63–75.

38. Russell JA. How much fluid resuscitation is optimal in septic shock? Crit Care 2012;16:146.

39. Stolmeijera R, ter Maatena JC, Zijlstrab JG, et al. Oxygen therapy for sepsis patients in the emergency department: a little less? Eur J Emerg Med 2014; 21(3):233–5.

40. Baskett A, Barton MH, Norton N, et al. Effect of pentoxifylline, flunixin meglu-mine, and their combination on a model of endotoxemia in horses. Am J Vet Res 1997;58(11):1291–9.

41. Bottoms GD, Fessler JF, Roesel OF, et al. Endotoxin-induced hemodynamic changes in ponies: effects of flunixin meglumine. Am J Vet Res 1981;42(9): 1514–8.
42. Bottoms GD, Templeton CB, Fessler JF, et al. Thromboxane, prostaglandin I2 (epoprostenol), and the hemodynamic changes in equine endotoxin shock. Am J Vet Res 1982;43(6):999–1002.
43. Ewert KM, Fessler JF, Templeton CB, et al. Endotoxin-induced hematologic and blood chemical changes in ponies: effects of flunixin meglumine, dexamethasone, and prednisolone. Am J Vet Res 1985;46(1):24–30.
44. Templeton CB, Bottoms GD, Fessler JF, et al. Endotoxin-induced hemodynamic and prostaglandin changes in ponies: effects of flunixin meglumine, dexamethasone, and prednisolone. Circ Shock 1987;23(4):231–40.
45. Fugler LA, Eades SC, Moore RM, et al. Plasma matrix metalloproteinase activity in horses after intravenous infusion of lipopolysaccharide and treatment with matrix metalloproteinase inhibitors. Am J Vet Res 2013;74(3):473–80.
46. Semrad SD, Hardee GE, Hardee MM, et al. Low dose flunixin meglumine: effects on eicosanoid production and clinical signs induced by experimental endotoxaemia in horses. Equine Vet J 1987;19(3):201–6.
47. Shuster R, Traub-Dargatz J, Baxter G. Survey of diplomates of the American College of Veterinary Internal Medicine and the American College of Veterinary Surgeons regarding clinical aspects and treatment of endotoxemia in horses. J Am Vet Med Assoc 1997;210(1):87–92.
48. Barton MH, Parviainen A, Norton N. Polymyxin B protects horses against induced endotoxaemia in vivo. Equine Vet J 2004;36(5):397–401.
49. Durando MM, MacKay RJ, Linda S, et al. Effects of polymyxin B and Salmonella typhimurium antiserum on horses given endotoxin intravenously. Am J Vet Res 1994;55(7):921–7.
50. MacKay RJ, Clark CK, Logdberg L, et al. Effect of a conjugate of polymyxin B-dextran 70 in horses with experimentally induced endotoxemia. Am J Vet Res 1999;60(1):68–75.
51. Sato K, Maekawa H, Sakurada M, et al. Direct hemoperfusion with polymyxin B immobilized fiber for abdominal sepsis in Europe. Surg Today 2011;41: 754–60.
52. Baldwin G, Alpert G, Caputo GL, et al. Effect of polymyxin B on experimental shock from meningococcal and Escherichia coli endotoxins. J Infect Dis 1991;164:542–9.
53. Haque KN, Pammi M. Pentoxifylline for treatment of sepsis and necrotizing enterocolitis in neonates. Cochrane Database Syst Rev 2011;(10):CD004205.
54. Harris E, Schulzke SM, Patole SK. Pentoxifylline in preterm neonates: a systematic review. Paediatr Drugs 2010;12(5):301–11.
55. Calandra T, Glauser MP, Schellekens J. Treatment of Gram-negative septic shock with human IgG antibody to Escherichia coli J5: a prospective, double-blind, randomized trial. J Infect Dis 1988;158:312–9.
56. Greenman RL, Schein RM, Martin MA, et al. A controlled clinical trial of E5 murine monoclonal IgM antibody to endotoxin in the treatment of Gramnegative sepsis. JAMA 1991;266:1097–102.
57. Mccloskey RV, Straube RC, Sanders C, et al. CHESS Trial Study Group. Treatment of septic shock with human monoclonal antibody HA-1A. Ann Intern Med 1994;121:1–5.
58. Prophylactic intravenous administration of standard immune globulin as compared with core-lipopolysaccharide immune globulin in patients at high

risk of postsurgical infection. The Intravenous Immunoglobulin Collaborative Study Group. N Engl J Med 1992;327:234–40.

59. Spier SJ, Lavoie JP, Cullor JS, et al. Protection against clinical endotoxemia in horses by using plasma containing antibody to an Rc mutant E. coli (J5). Circ Shock 1989;28(3):235–48.

60. Van den Berghe G, Wouters P, Weekers F, et al. Intensive insulin therapy in critically ill patients. N Engl J Med 2001;345:1359–67.

61. Forbes NC, Anders N. Does tight glycemic control improve outcomes in pediatric patients undergoing surgery and/or those with critical illness? Int J Gen Med 2013;7:1–11.

62. Hollis AR, Furr MO, Magdesian KG, et al. Blood glucose concentrations in critically ill neonatal foals. J Vet Intern Med 2008;22(5):1223–7.

63. NICE-SUGAR Study Investigators, Finfer S, Chittock DR, et al. Intensive versus conventional glucose control in critically ill patients. N Engl J Med 2009;360: 1283–97.

64. Gold J, Divers T, Barton M, et al. Plasma adrenocorticotropin, cortisol, and adrenocorticotropin/cortisol ratios in septic and normal-term foals. J Vet Intern Med 2007;21:791–6.

65. Hurcombe S, Toribio R, Slovis N, et al. Blood arginine vasopressin, adrenocorticotropin hormone, and cortisol concentrations at admission in septic and critically ill foals and their association with survival. J Vet Intern Med 2008;22: 639–47.

66. Wong D, Vo D, Alcott C, et al. Baseline plasma cortisol and ACTH concentrations and response to low dose ACTH stimulation testing in ill foals. J Am Med Assoc 2009;234:126–32.

67. Hart KA, Slovis NM, Barton MH. Hypothalamic-pituitary-adrenal axis dysfunction in hospitalized neonatal foals. J Vet Intern Med 2009;23:901–12.

68. Hart KA, Barton MH, Ferguson DC, et al. Serum free cortisol fraction in healthy and septic neonatal foals. J Vet Intern Med 2011;25:345–55.

69. Armengou L, Jose-Cunilleras E, Ríos J, et al. Metabolic and endocrine profiles in sick neonatal foals are related to survival. J Vet Intern Med 2013;27(3):567–75.

70. Menon K, Ward RE, Lawson ML, et al. A prospective multicenter study of adrenal function in critically ill children. Am J Respir Crit Care Med 2010;182:246–51.

71. Annane D, Sebille V, Charpentier C, et al. Effect of treatment with low doses of hydrocortisone and fludrocortisone on mortality in patients with septic shock. JAMA 2002;288:862–71.

72. Sprung CL, Annane D, Keh D, et al. Hydrocortisone therapy for patients with septic shock. N Engl J Med 2008;358:111–24.

73. Markovitz BP, Goodman DM, Watson RS, et al. A retrospective cohort study of prognostic factors associated with outcome in pediatric severe sepsis: what is the role of steroids? Pediatr Crit Care Med 2005;6:270–4.

74. Zimmerman JJ. A history of adjunctive glucocorticoid treatment for pediatric sepsis: moving beyond steroid pulp fiction toward evidence-based medicine. Pediatr Crit Care Med 2007;8:530–9.

75. Smith CM. Origin and uses of primum non nocere–above all, do no harm! J Clin Pharmacol 2005;45(4):371–7.

Is it the Systemic Inflammatory Response Syndrome or Endotoxemia in Horses with Colic?

James N. Moore, DVM, PhD[a,b,*], Michel L. Vandenplas, PhD[c]

KEYWORDS

- Lipopolysaccharide • Endotoxin • Systemic inflammation • Innate immunity
- Toll-like receptors

KEY POINTS

- Endotoxins are the structural components of the outer cell wall of gram-negative bacteria that are perceived as the worst of bad news by the innate immune system.
- The term endotoxemia is commonly used by veterinarians to describe the clinical status of horses in which circulatory system function and tissue perfusion are impaired.
- The systemic inflammatory response syndrome (SIRS) describes the body's response to infection and trauma whereby there is evidence of organ dysfunction and failure.
- While the innate immune system serves as the first line of defense against microbial invasion, it also is the source of inflammatory mediators that result in SIRS.

INTRODUCTION

Speak with equine practitioners about problems they face treating horses that have colic and invariably the term endotoxemia will be used. Furthermore, endotoxemia will be mentioned as it relates to the development of acute laminitis and other complications, including jugular vein thrombosis. In most of these instances, the physiologic changes typically associated with endotoxemia are alterations in heart and respiratory rates, mucous membrane color, and capillary refill time. Because the term endotoxemia actually refers to the presence of bacterial endotoxins in the circulation, it has been suggested that other terms should be used instead to describe the clinical status

The authors have nothing to disclose.
[a] Department of Large Animal Medicine, College of Veterinary Medicine, University of Georgia, 501 DW Brooks Drive, Athens, GA 30602, USA; [b] Department of Physiology and Pharmacology, College of Veterinary Medicine, University of Georgia, 501 DW Brooks Drive, Athens, GA 30602, USA; [c] Ross University School of Veterinary Medicine, PO Box 334, Basseterre, Saint Kitts, West Indies
* Corresponding author. Department of Large Animal Medicine, College of Veterinary Medicine, University of Georgia, Athens, GA 30602.
E-mail address: jmoore@uga.edu

Vet Clin Equine 30 (2014) 337–351
http://dx.doi.org/10.1016/j.cveq.2014.04.003   vetequine.theclinics.com
0749-0739/14/$ – see front matter © 2014 Elsevier Inc. All rights reserved.

of these horses. Of these, the term that has received the greatest interest is the systemic inflammatory response syndrome (SIRS). The goal of this article is to provide the information needed for the reader to determine which is more appropriate, and answer the question: Is it SIRS or endotoxemia in horses with colic?

SIRS

More than 20 years ago, human physicians wrestled with how best to define the different clinical scenarios they faced with severely ill patients who were at increased risk of developing life-threatening complications or dying. In their experience, many of their patients with trauma, ischemia, pancreatitis, or tissue injury exhibited clinical signs identical to those associated with infections, but lacked identifiable sources of infection or bacteria in their bloodstream. In an effort to describe the situation in these patients they coined the phrase systemic inflammatory response syndrome or SIRS, and identified the criteria that had to be met for a patient to have SIRS.[1] These criteria included specific changes in body temperature, heart rate, respiratory rate, and white blood cell count; at least 2 of these changes had to exist before a patient had SIRS.

Many horses with colic and neonatal critically ill foals exhibit clinical signs similar to those described for SIRS. As a result, at least 2 sets of criteria have been proposed to define SIRS in horses and foals. In a study of critically ill foals presented to a teaching hospital clinic for evaluation and treatment, the presence of SIRS was based on meeting at least 2 of the following criteria: leukocytosis, leukopenia or greater than 10% immature band neutrophils, hyperthermia or hypothermia, tachycardia, tachypnea, and evidence of sepsis.[2] More than 40% of the foals evaluated had a diagnosis of SIRS. Using a slightly modified set of criteria (leukocytosis, leukopenia or >10% immature band neutrophils, hyperthermia, tachycardia, and tachypnea), Epstein and colleagues[3] determined that nearly 30% of adult horses presented for evaluation and treatment of colic had evidence of SIRS (**Box 1**).

Thus far, the diseases that have been associated with the presence of SIRS in neonatal foals primarily are bacteremia, local bacterial infections (eg, umbilical infection, pneumonia, septic arthritis, and pyelonephritis), and perinatal asphyxia syndrome.[2] Similarly, the diseases that have been associated with SIRS in adult horses are restricted to those involving the gastrointestinal tract,[3] including the inflammatory intestinal diseases (eg, enteritis and colitis) and strangulating obstructions (eg, pedunculated lipomas, large colon volvulus, and small intestinal entrapments or strangulations). It also has been suggested that SIRS and sepsis-related laminitis occur in horses with pleuropneumonia, septic endometritis, and carbohydrate overload of the gastrointestinal tract,[4] although specific studies designed to document the occurrence of SIRS in these diseases have yet to be reported. Furthermore, the clinical

---

Box 1
Criteria for a diagnosis of SIRS (at least 2 required)

- Abnormality in leukocyte count or distribution (leukopenia, leukocytosis, or >10% band neutrophils)
- Hyperthermia or hypothermia
- Tachycardia
- Tachypnea
- Evidence of sepsis in foals

manifestations of pneumonia in foals caused by *Rhodococcus equi*, a gram-positive organism, are consistent with the presence of SIRS.[5]

THE INNATE IMMUNE SYSTEM

The first line of defense against the microorganisms that cause disease is the innate immune system. In keeping with its name, the innate immune system is present in all individuals and responds quickly to the pathogen, most often within minutes. In evolutionary terms, it is also the oldest form of immunity, existing in species from plants to mammals. In most instances, these immune responses are sufficient to prevent invasion of the tissues by the pathogens and the development of infections. However, the innate immune system does not provide long-term memory or selective specificity against pathogens; this responsibility is left to the adaptive immune system.

One of the primary functions of the innate immune system is to recruit phagocytes, primarily neutrophils and mononuclear phagocytes, to the area of tissue damage; this is achieved through the production and release of chemical mediators called cytokines. In doing so, these cytokines, in addition to other mediators released or expressed by the recruited inflammatory cells, cause the typical clinical findings associated with inflammation, namely localized redness, heat, swelling, and pain. These findings are due to local physiologic changes, including dilation of blood vessels, extravasation of plasma proteins and fluid, and a reduction in the threshold for stimulation of nociceptors that sense pain.

The most rapidly functioning components of the innate immune system are specific soluble factors that exist in the circulation and extracellular fluid, or are secreted by epithelial cells. The purpose of these factors is to kill the pathogens or at least reduce the likelihood that they will establish an active infection. These factors include enzymes, such as lysozyme, that digest the bacterial cell walls, the complement system that identifies and targets pathogens for lysis and phagocytosis, and antimicrobial peptides that cause direct lysis of the bacterial cell membranes. A more slowly acting component of the innate immune system is the recognition of microbial molecules, called pathogen-associated molecular patterns (PAMPs) by cellular receptors. The most notable of these PAMPs are endotoxin (ie, lipopolysaccharide [LPS]), flagellin, peptidoglycan, lipoteichoic acid, double-stranded viral RNA, and unmethylated CpG motifs.[6] Binding of these PAMPs to their respective receptors results in activation of the cells and initiation of additional responses designed to combat the pathogens and eliminate them from the body. The critical nature of the innate immune system is exemplified by the deleterious effects of genetic abnormalities that result in the absence or dysfunction of 1 or more components of the system.

PATTERN-RECOGNITION RECEPTORS AND THEIR ROLE IN EQUINE SIRS

Innate immune responses to infection are mediated through distinct classes of receptors expressed on the surface of cells or in intracellular compartments, including: toll-like receptors (TLRs); nucleotide-binding leucine-rich repeat containing receptors; retinoic acid–inducible gene-1–like receptors; C-type lectins; and Absent-in-melanoma-like receptors. The structure and function of these receptors were reviewed in detail recently by Bryant and Monie.[7] Of these receptors, only the TLRs have been studied in equine cells, either by quantifying expression of the genes that encode the individual TLR proteins themselves (ie, TLR1–TLR10) in different equine tissues and cells, by monitoring the responses of equine leukocytes exposed to stimuli that activate specific TLRs in other species, by heterologous expression of specific TLRs (eg, TLR4, TLR8, and TLR9) in HEK cells, or by identifying equine TLR gene homologues (eg, TLR7).[8–15] Although the precise complement of equine TLRs has not been determined, 10 have been identified by one or other means, a number similar to that found in humans.[7] However, it is known that the complement, function, and number of TLRs can differ between more distantly related species (**Box 2**).[7]

TLR4 AND ITS INTERACTIONS WITH LPS

The most widely studied TLR is TLR4 which, together with its accessory receptor, MD-2, responds to monomeric endotoxins. Naturally occurring LPS, a vital component of the cell walls of gram-negative bacteria, is made up of 3 distinct structural parts.[16] The outermost polysaccharide O antigen domain of LPS is a repetitive glycan polymer that varies from strain to strain and is a target for recognition by host antibodies; this is connected to a core domain that consists of less variant oligosaccharides. The innermost component of LPS, Lipid A, is a phosphorylated glucosamine disaccharide attached to up to 6 hydrophobic fatty acids. Lipid A anchors the LPS molecule into the bacterial cell membrane, is responsible for many of the toxic effects of gram-negative bacteria, and is the smallest ligand recognized by TLR4/MD-2. Having both hydrophobic lipid and hydrophilic sugar moieties, LPS forms micelles in aqueous solutions. These features of LPS are important for the regulation of its movement in the circulation and its interaction with cells. Binding of LPS to TLR4 initiates cell-signaling cascades (see later discussion), activation of the cell, and the synthesis of mediators associated with inflammation. Equine cells, specifically monocytes, are highly sensitive to the presence of LPS, having a half-maximal effective concentration (EC_{50}) of 0.013 to 0.030 ng/mL for *Escherichia coli* LPS for the release of tumor necrosis factor α (TNFα) and expression of tissue factor.[13] This low EC_{50} demonstrates the high sensitivity of horses to the presence of LPS in the circulation.

SIGNALING PATHWAYS INITIATED BY TLR4 ACTIVATION

Before interacting with TLR4, monomers of LPS must be released from the micelles that have formed in the plasma. This process is facilitated by a specific serum protein called LPS-binding protein.[17] The excised LPS monomers are then transferred to a receptor called CD14, which exists as attached to either the surface of myeloid cells by a phosphatidylinositol linkage or a soluble protein in plasma. After it binds to CD14, LPS can then interact with TLR4 and its coreceptor protein, MD-2. TLR4 receptors then come together to initiate the activation of discrete intracellular pathways. Based on information from the extensive work that has been performed using cells of other species, TLR4 activation leads to TLR/interleukin (IL)-1 receptor-associated protein (TIRAP)-dependent recruitment of the MyD88 adaptor protein.[18,19] Recruitment of

| Box 2 |
| Examples of ligands for equine toll-like receptors |

TLR1/2	Triacyl lipopeptides (synthetic analogue, Pam_3CSK_4)
TLR2	Lipoproteins, peptidoglycan, lipoteichoic acids
TLR3	Double-stranded viral RNA (synthetic analogue, poly I:C)
TLR4	Lipopolysaccharide
TLR5	Flagellin
TLR6/2	Zymosan
TLR7	Single-strand RNA, imidazoquinolines
TLR8	Single-strand RNA, imidazoquinolines
TLR9	Unmethylated CpG DNA
TLR10	Undetermined

MyD88 has 2 effects that occur in the cytosol: (1) degradation of IκB and subsequent activation of the transcription factor nuclear factor κB (NF-κB), and (2) phosphorylation of the mitogen-activated protein kinases and activation of additional transcription factors. NF-κB and the other transcription factors then move into the nucleus, where they bind to specific sites in the promoter regions of genes associated with inflammation. This binding induces the transcription of a variety of genes, including those for proinflammatory mediators such as TNFα and IL-1β. This early set of events primarily leads to the release of proinflammatory mediators.

After a delay, TLR4 receptors activated by LPS recruit 2 other adaptor molecules, called TRIF and TRAM.[19,20] These steps lead not only to a secondary, delayed activation of NF-κB and mitogen-activated protein kinases but also to activation and nuclear translocation of the transcription factor interferon regulatory factor 3 (IRF3). Once inside the nucleus, IRF3 promotes expression of the interferon (IFN)α/β gene and subsequent induction of IFN-responsive genes, such as CCL5 (RANTES) and IP-10. The end result of these processes is an increased expression of the gene encoding the anti-inflammatory mediator, IL-10. Thus, whereas the MyD88 pathway promotes the production of proinflammatory mediators, the TRIF pathway is viewed as being anti-inflammatory in nature.[20] Based on studies using human dendritic cells, switching occurs between the MyD88 and TRIF signaling pathways (**Fig. 1**). This switching is controlled by the delta isoform of phosphatidylinositol-3-OH kinase (PI(3)K), with activated PI(3)Kδ leading to the release of TIRAP and MyD88 from the TLR4s in the cell membrane.[21] As a result of these and other processes (eg, calcium mobilization), TLR4 then becomes internalized in endosomes where it is able to interact with TRAM-associated TRIF.[20] The time required for TLR4 internalization helps account for the delayed activation of the TRIF pathway relative to that of the MyD88 pathway.

OTHER EQUINE TLRS AND THEIR PAMPS

The TLR that primarily recognizes components of gram-positive bacteria is TLR2. When bound by one of its bacterial ligands, TLR2 forms heterodimers with either TLR1 or TLR6, which results in activation of only the MyD88 pathway. Ligands for TLR2 include peptidoglycan, mostly from the cell walls of gram-positive bacteria but to a lesser extent from gram-negative bacteria, mycobacterial lipoarabinomannan, lipoteichoic acid, lipoproteins, and yeast zymozan.[6,7] Of particular interest to equine medicine, VapA, one of the proteins encoded by the large virulence plasmid in *R equi,* is a ligand for TLR2, indicating that TLR2-mediated responses to *R equi* could be an important contributor to equine pulmonary disease.[22] Thus, at present TLR2 seems to be the most promiscuous of the characterized TLRs in terms of the number of different types of microbial ligands it recognizes.

In cultured equine monocytes, the synthetic TLR2 ligand, PAM_3CSK_4, induces expression of the genes for TNFα and IL-1β, but not for the TRIF-dependent genes (specifically CCL5, IFNβ, and IP-10).[13] Thus, like cells from other mammals, TLR2 in equine monocytes signals only through MyD88. The EC_{50} of PAM_3CSK_4 that results in the release of TNFα and expression of tissue factor by these cells is 1.0 to 4.7 ng/mL.[13] These concentrations are orders of magnitude higher than those required for initiation of these same responses by LPS. In the case of rhodococcal VapA protein, the local concentrations of the ligand at the site of bacterial infection in the lung may be far more important than concentrations of VapA as it is disseminated in the circulation.

The TLRs also are important in the recognition of viruses, with this function being the responsibility of TLR3. Poly I:C, a mimetic of double-stranded viral RNA, activates

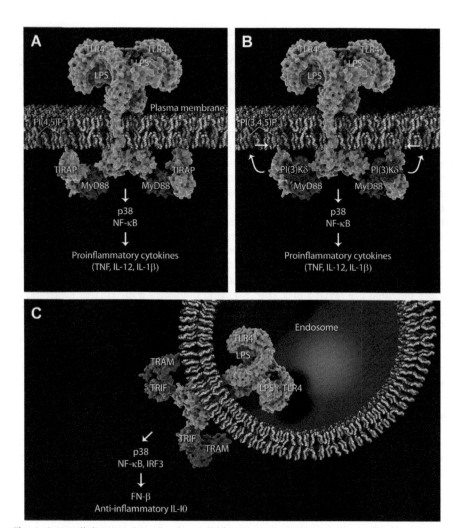

Fig. 1. Intracellular signaling distal to toll-like receptor 4 (TLR4). TLR4 signaling occurs in 3 essential steps.[20] (*A*) Binding of lipopolysaccharide (LPS) to the extracellular domain of TLR4 causes receptor dimerization, recruitment of MyD88 to phosphatidylinositol(4,5)bisphosphate (PI(4,5)P$_2$)-associated TLR/interleukin-1 receptor–associated protein (TIRAP), and the induction of proinflammatory responses. (*B*) Through the action of phosphatidylinositol-3-OH kinase δ (PI(3)Kδ), the membrane anchor of TIRAP, PI(4,5)P$_2$ becomes phosphorylated to produce phosphatidylinositol(3,4,5)triphosphate (PI(3,4,5)P$_3$), thereby causing the release of TIRAP and MyD88. (*C*) As a consequence TLR4 becomes internalized, where it associates with the TRAM/TRIF complex, allowing for initiation of anti-inflammatory responses. FN-β, interferon-β; IL, interleukin; IRF3, interferon regulatory factor 3; NF-κB, nuclear factor κB; TNF, tumor necrosis factor. (Illustrations by Brad Gilleland; *courtesy of* the University of Georgia, Athens, GA.)

cultured equine monocytes dose-dependently and results in expression of genes (IFNβ, CCL5, and IL-10) that depend on involvement of TRIF.[13] In other mammals TLR3, located in endosomes, signals solely through the TRIF pathway. Because of the intracellular location of TLR3, the EC$_{50}$ of poly I:C required for expression of IFNβ by equine monocytes has not been accurately determined, but appears to be high (>μg/mL range). Although many of the retroviruses responsible for equine viral diseases (eg, equine infectious anemia virus, equine arteritis virus, and eastern equine encephalitis virus) have single-stranded RNA genomes, regions of their genomes can be double-stranded and thus potentially could act as TLR3 ligands.[23,24] However, this suggestion is tempered by the finding that equine arteritis virus signals through MyD88 to NF-κB activation.[25] It is also known that viruses can have a major effect on TLR responses, as many viruses have the ability to regulate NF-κB activity.[26] For example, a West Nile virus factor, NS1, can block TLR3-mediated activation of NF-κB and IRF3.[27] It is clear that more research is required to address the effects of viral infection on initiation and modulation of TLR-mediated innate immune responses in horses.

As occurs in other species, bacterial flagellin is recognized by TLR5 in equine cells. Equine neutrophils produce reactive oxygen species (ROS) in response to flagellin, with an EC_{50} of 20 to 40 ng/mL.[14] These concentrations are approximately 10-fold greater than those associated with activation of monocytes by the TLR2 ligand, PAM_3CSK_4.[13] Similarly to TLR2 and most other TLRs, TLR5 signaling only through the MyD88 pathway and in equine neutrophils leads to the induction of TNFα and cyclooxygenase-2 gene expression.[14]

Equine TLR8 in reporter gene assays responds to ligands in a similar fashion to other higher mammals (eg, humans and cows), but distinct from rodent TLR8 ligand responses,[28] owing to the loss of 5 amino acids in the ectodomain of rodent TLR8. The natural ligand for this receptor is single-strand viral RNA. Equine TLR9, as found in other species, responds to CpG DNA, but these responses have not been examined in any great detail in equine cells. It is interesting that while equine neutrophil responses to TLR9 activation include release of ROS and the induction of IFNγ, IL-8, and IL-12 gene expression, TNFα gene expression was significantly reduced by 4 hours after stimulation.[29] TLR8 and TLR9 are closely related and therefore have overlapping responses to synthetic ligands, and, similar to TLR3, have an intracellular location complicating EC_{50} determination.[28]

Thus far the ligand-induced cellular responses of other TLRs known to be expressed by equine cells have not been characterized, and their potential contribution to SIRS in horses is unknown.

MEDIATORS RELEASED VIA TLR ACTIVATION AND THEIR PHYSIOLOGIC EFFECTS

The consequence of TLR activation is the induction and release of proinflammatory mediators from peripheral blood monocytes and neutrophils. These mediators include prostaglandins, cytokines, procoagulant activity (ie, tissue factor), and ROS.[13,30] The timing and magnitude of these cellular responses is important to the establishment of SIRS. For example, induction of TNFα gene expression is rapid and transient (1 hour after stimulation), induction of IL-1β gene expression is sustained for a longer time interval (for up to 20 hours after stimulation) and induction of IL-6 expression is delayed and sustained (from 4 to 20 hours).[13] The proinflammatory mediators cause a secondary sequence of events mediated through cellular receptors on adjacent cells. These secondary events are in part responsible for the clinical symptoms observed in horses with colic, including abdominal pain, tachycardia, alterations in borborygmi, and increased rectal temperature. The underlying purpose for the immediate proinflammatory responses of the innate immune system to microbes is to kill and remove invading pathogens. It is the robust activation and overproduction of these mediators that is deleterious to the host animal. Consequently, cellular responses also include the production of anti-inflammatory cytokines (eg, IL-10) and other mediators (eg, adenosine), in addition to downregulation of TLR receptors through receptor-mediated endocytosis and degradation of elements of the intracellular signaling pathways distal to the receptor. This latter process, known as tolerance, causes a delayed induction of TLR gene expression to reestablish the TLRs and restore cellular responsiveness.[31] In equine monocytes, LPS and PAM_3CSK_4, bacterial components that signal initially through TLR4 and TLR2, respectively, and then through MyD88, cause induction of both TLR4 and TLR2 genes.[32] By contrast, poly I:C–induced activation of the TRIF pathway through TLR3 does not cause induction of TLR4 and TLR2 expression. Thus, the balance between proinflammatory and anti-inflammatory mediators also determines the fate of the host innate immune system response. In horses, this frequently culminates in SIRS.

DIFFERENCES IN RESPONSES OF EQUINE CELLS TO TLR ACTIVATION
Responses of Equine TLR4 to LPS

In contrast to the LPS-induced responses in other mammalian species, LPS activation of TLR4 in equine monocytes leads only to the engagement of the MyD88 pathway.[13] This eventuality is illustrated by the rapid and transient induction of TNFα gene expression, the rapid and sustained IL-1β gene expression, and the slower but sustained activation of IL-6 gene expression induced by LPS in equine peripheral blood monocytes. Expression of these 3 genes is the hallmark of MyD88 activation. By contrast, even high concentrations of LPS fail to induce expression of either CCL5 or IFNβ, hallmarks of gene expression governed by the TRIF/IRF3 pathway.[13] Interestingly the equine TLR4 responses to LPS are very similar to those induced through activation of the MyD88 pathway by TLR2 ligands, and distinct from those induced through the TRIF-dependent pathway by activation of TLR3.[13] Noteworthy are the large differences in the time required to induce IL-10 gene expression and the magnitude of this response by activation of these 3 different TLRs. Although activation of either TLR2 or TLR4 leads to induction of IL-10 gene expression, the magnitude of response is far greater for activation of TLR3. This fact is particularly important given that engagement of the TRIF pathway is regarded as being anti-inflammatory in nature, whereas the MyD88 pathway is responsible for inducing a proinflammatory state (see **Fig. 1**).[20] Switching of TLR4 signaling between MyD88 and TRIF is controlled through the action of PI(3)Kδ. This switching event appears to be absent in equine monocytes.[13] Given the low EC_{50} required for LPS to induce expression of proinflammatory cytokine genes in equine monocytes, the fact that TLR4 in equine monocytes signals only through MyD88, and the lack of induction of TRIF-dependent anti-inflammatory cytokines by equine TLR4, the proinflammatory responses of equine monocytes to LPS may be far stronger than those occurring in other animal species.

Agonist/Antagonist LPS Responses

In addition to the differences in the intracellular signaling pathways used by TLR4 in equine monocytes from those used by TLR4 in other animal species, equine TLR4 also responds differently to specific types of LPS in comparison with that of TLR4 from other species. For example, LPS isolated from *Rhodobacter sphaeroides* antagonizes the proinflammatory effects of *E coli* LPS in human and murine cells, but induces proinflammatory responses via TLR4 in equine cells.[10] Similarly, the LPS derivative, Lipid IV_A, a compound that acts as an antagonist of *E coli* LPS in human cells, is an agonist in equine cells.[33] Synthetic E5531, a compound developed for the treatment of endotoxemia based on the structure of *R sphaeroides* lipid A, is similar to its parent LPS, an antagonist of *E coli* LPS in human cells but an agonist in equine cells.[34] However, E5564, a synthetic compound with subtle structural differences from E5531, acts as a TLR4 antagonist in both human and equine cells.[35] Thus, slight differences in LPS structure can contribute markedly to the outcome of TLR4 responses in different mammalian species.

Equine-Specific Cellular Responses to Flagellin

As described earlier, flagellin, the ligand for TLR5, induces proinflammatory responses in equine neutrophils.[14] However, flagellin does not activate equine peripheral blood monocytes, as the expression of surface TLR5 in these cells is extremely low.[14] By contrast, monocytes from all other mammalian species (eg, humans, mice, cattle) studied to date respond strongly to flagellin and do so through TLR5.[14] This finding provides additional support to the notion that cellular innate immune responses to PAMPs in horses are different from those of other animals.

Important aspects of equine innate system responses

- Exquisitely high sensitivity of equine cells to LPS
- SIRS is not only associated with LPS stimulation; it occurs with gram-positive organisms (eg, *R equi*)
- LPS stimulation of equine monocytes selectively involves the MyD88 pathway, resulting in proinflammatory effects
- Compounds that function as LPS antagonists in other species activate equine cells
- Flagellin selectively activates neutrophils in horses, not monocytes

---

THE FOCUS ON ENDOTOXEMIA

The focus on endotoxins is not new. In fact, endotoxins have been the focus of studies since the early 1890s when Richard Pfeiffer, a colleague of Robert Koch in Germany, identified heat-stable "toxins linked to the bacterial body substance" that caused circulatory shock and death in laboratory animals.[36] Before the end of that decade, Coley[37] reported "antitumor" activity associated with infections, and initiated clinical studies using a combination of bacterial organisms. These toxins were administered to patients with cancer in the United States from the early 1920s until 1963. Interest in endotoxins increased in the 1940s, when it was determined that the heat-stable toxins were, in fact, LPS, and it became possible to purify them from bacterial culture supernatants. During this time the fields of chemistry, biochemistry, and immunology were beginning to overlap, and studies were performed in which the in vivo effects of LPS were more fully characterized, the phenomenon of endotoxin tolerance was identified, and the structure of lipid A was determined.[36] Throughout this period it was assumed that the lipid-rich nature of endotoxins somehow allowed them to intercalate themselves into cell membranes and cause damage to the host. During the same period one very important discovery received relatively little attention, namely that a strain of mice had been produced that resulted in the inheritance of resistance to experimental administration of endotoxins.[38] Clearly this finding should have caused more researchers to consider other mechanisms by which LPS interacts with cells. However, the concept of endotoxins as "toxins" that by themselves damaged host cells was entrenched in the literature, and the focus on endotoxemia was strong.

In the mid-1960s Carroll, Schalm, and Wheat performed the first study evaluating the effects of endotoxin in a single horse, followed in the 1970s by a series of studies in which different dosages and routes of administration of LPS were evaluated in ponies.[39] The concentrations of LPS used in these studies (180 μg/kg) were extrapolated from those used in other species, and were found to be excessive. These studies were followed by others in which much lower dosages of LPS were evaluated, in an effort to more closely simulate the effects of endotoxemia identified in clinical patients with gastrointestinal diseases. By necessity, the focus of these early studies was to characterize the effects of experimental endotoxemia, primarily documenting the cardiopulmonary responses that occurred as a result of administration of LPS, either as a bolus injection or slow infusion given intravenously, or as single or intermittent injections given intraperitoneally.

In the late 1970s, two things happened simultaneously to change the way these studies were performed: first, the discovery of arachidonic acid metabolism and the role of prostaglandins in pain and inflammation, and second, the release of flunixin meglumine as an analgesic for horses with colic. The combination of these two findings made possible the realization that the ill effects of endotoxins were not due to the endotoxins themselves but were the result of the body's response. These discoveries were followed fairly closely by the development of radioimmunoassays that allowed researchers to monitor changes in plasma concentrations of the stable metabolites of individual arachidonic acid metabolites in response to administration of LPS and the effects of flunixin meglumine thereon. The availability of these assays made it possible to recognize which physiologic responses to LPS were associated with arachidonic acid metabolism, and which were not.

The focus of the research community quickly switched from arachidonic acid metabolism to TNF in the 1980s. Initially thought to exist as 2 related factors synthesized by macrophages, named TNFα and TNFβ, it is now known that there are 19 members of the TNF superfamily of cytokines that are involved in inflammation, cellular proliferation, and apoptosis (ie, programmed cell death).[40] Once it became possible to detect TNFα in serum samples, this became the primary focus of work on experimental endotoxemia and in clinical cases of colic.[41]

The next decade of research focused largely on the identification and characterization of the interleukins, a large family of cytokines that helps initiate and modulate cellular responses during inflammation and immune system responses, and on tissue factor, a cell-surface response to LPS that directly linked mononuclear phagocytes with the coagulation cascade. The availability of laboratory assays to detect these inflammatory mediators made it possible to monitor the effects of experimental endotoxemia and to characterize their role in horses with colic.[42] During this period, additional studies were performed in horses using short-term infusions of much smaller doses of LPS (30 ng/kg) in an effort to induce physiologic responses that more closely mimic those seen in clinical cases.[43]

In 1997, Janeway, Medzhitov, and Beutler extended Hoffman's previous work on the role of toll receptors in fungal infections in fruit flies to mammals, and in so doing changed the landscape of research on infection and immunity. These investigators identified TLR4 and showed that it functions as the cell-surface receptor for LPS. Subsequent work, largely by Akira, resulted in the identification of most members of the TLR family of receptors described herein. Furthermore, Hoshino and colleagues[44] soon determined that the strain of LPS-resistant mice described some 50 years earlier had a mutation in the TLR4 gene that accounted for their lack of response to LPS.

The complexity of the host response to LPS has most recently been elucidated through the use of quantitative reverse transcription–polymerase chain reaction. Rather than monitoring changes in circulating concentrations of a few inflammatory mediators, this approach makes it possible to simultaneously monitor changes in the expression of a variety of genes in cells. This approach has been used to evaluate the response of cells isolated from horses with colic and horses after carbohydrate overload of the gastrointestinal tract.[45,46]

DETECTION OF LPS

In the 1970s, Bang and Levin developed the first laboratory test that allowed for the detection of small amounts of endotoxins in body fluids. This assay arose from studies Bang was performing on the circulation of hemolymph in the horseshoe crab, Limulus polyphemus. During one of his studies, 1 of the crabs died of an infection caused by a Vibrio organism, and one of the principal findings was that essentially all of the crab's hemolymph had clotted. This discovery led to a series of studies that culminated in the 2 scientists determining that the same effects on hemolymph could be produced with endotoxins isolated from gram-negative bacteria, and the development of the Limulus amebocyte lysate assay. Subsequent improvements to this assay that have incorporated the use of a chromogenic substrate now allow the detection of extremely small concentrations of endotoxin in plasma. The results of several clinical studies performed using this assay indicate that approximately 30% of adult horses with colic and 50% of critically ill neonatal foals presented to veterinary teaching hospitals have LPS in their circulation.[47–49] When LPS is detected, typically it is in horses with diseases having either inflammation or ischemia in their pathogenesis. In one study, the likelihood that LPS would be detected in the circulation was significantly higher for horses with tachycardia, increased packed cell volume, and clinical disease/surgical findings typically associated with translocation of LPS from the gastrointestinal tract into the circulation.[49] The potential contribution of other PAMPs to the development of SIRS in horses has not been investigated. In humans, bacterial DNA has been detected in the circulation of patients with SIRS.[50] Similarly, administration of flagellin to mice causes a severe form of acute lung inflammation, and both flagellin and antibodies directed against flagellin have been detected in serum samples from human patients with Crohn disease.[51–53]

SIRS OR ENDOTOXEMIA?

Although the term endotoxemia seems to be firmly entrenched in the veterinary lexicon, the data indicate that the clinical signs associated with inflammatory or ischemic diseases ultimately are the result of the inflammatory mediators synthesized by the horse's cells rather than by the presence of endotoxins in circulation. This conclusion is further supported by similar clinical signs that can be evident in animals with infections caused by gram-positive bacteria (eg, R equi), and the likelihood that bacterial components other than LPS enter the circulation in animals with intestinal inflammation or ischemia, as shown in humans. Thus, SIRS would be a more accurate term to describe what many now refer to as clinical endotoxemia. It is important, however, to keep in mind that the concentrations of LPS required to initiate systemic inflammatory responses in horse cells are orders of magnitude lower than those required for other bacterial components, and the impact of LPS on the animal's status cannot be overlooked.

TREATMENT
Current Treatment Approach

At present, the mainstays of treating affected horses and foals that either have been evaluated experimentally or have not fallen out of favor over time are intravenous fluid replacement, nonsteroidal anti-inflammatory drugs (NSAIDs), and polymyxin B.[54] Other therapeutic approaches that have been used, but either lack experimentally derived data to support their continued use or have been replaced by other therapies, include plasma containing antibodies directed against the lipid A moiety in LPS, dimethyl sulfoxide, heparin, and pentoxifylline.

Most commonly, isotonic, polyionic electrolyte solutions are used for fluid therapy; in some instances, particularly for long-term use, additional potassium is provided by adding KCl to the solution. When dictated by the severity of disease, rapid restoration of circulating fluid volume can be facilitated by the administration of hypertonic saline, and colloids may be used to help retain fluids within the vascular space in hypoproteinemic animals.

Based on their ability to prevent the production of prostaglandins by inhibiting arachidonic acid metabolism, NSAIDs are commonly used in affected animals. The most commonly used agent is flunixin meglumine, which often is administered at either 0.25 mg/kg or 1.1 mg/kg. The rationale for the use of the lower dose is based on an early study in which many of the ill effects of experimental endotoxin administration were prevented by this dose, and the concern about potentially masking clinical signs associated with intestinal ischemia at the higher dose. As the higher dose recommended by the manufacturer prevents additional effects of LPS, many clinicians prefer to administer this dose at 12-hour intervals.

The cationic polypeptide antimicrobial, polymyxin B, binds avidly to the lipid A moiety of LPS. For this reason it has been studied experimentally in horses administered LPS, and often is administered to animals at increased risk for translocation of LPS across the damaged intestine or exhibiting signs of SIRS. A wide range of doses are used in clinical cases, very often at or near the 5000 U/kg used in an in vivo study of experimental endotoxemia.[43] It is reasonable to question the effectiveness of this therapy once signs of SIRS are present.

Caution Regarding Extrapolating Future Treatments to Horses

Translational medical studies must be interpreted with care. What's good for the goose is not necessarily good for the gander or, in this case, what works well in one species may have adverse effects in the horse. This view is substantiated by the findings that natural and synthetic lipid A–based compounds function as LPS antagonists in humans, but as agonists in horses.[34] Similarly, the fact that changes in gene expression during SIRS are different in mice and humans may explain why many drugs developed for the treatment of SIRS based on studies performed in mice fail to yield beneficial effects in human clinical trials.[55] Consequently, drugs that are effective in studies performed in laboratory animals may not have a positive outcome for the management of SIRS in horses.

REFERENCES

1. Bone RC, Balk RA, Cerra FB, et al. Definitions for sepsis and organ failure and guidelines for the use of innovative therapies in sepsis. Chest 1992;101: 1644–55.
2. Corley KT, Donaldson LL, Furr MO. Arterial lactate concentration, hospital survival, sepsis and SIRS in critically ill neonatal foals. Equine Vet J 2005;37: 53–9.
3. Epstein KL, Brainard BM, Gomez-Ibanez SE, et al. Thrombelastography in horses with acute gastrointestinal disease. J Vet Intern Med 2011;25(2):307–14.
4. Belknap JK, Black SJ. Sepsis-related laminitis. Equine Vet J 2012;44:738–40.
5. Giguere S, Cohen ND, Chaffin MK, et al. *Rhodococcus equi*: Clinical manifestations, virulence and immunity. J Vet Intern Med 2011;25:1221–30.
6. Werners AH, Bryant CE. Pattern recognition receptors in equine endotoxaemia and sepsis. Equine Vet J 2012;44:490–8.

7. Bryant CE, Monie TP. Mice, men and the relatives: cross-species studies underpin innate immunity. Open Biol 2012;2(4):120015.
8. Astakhova NM, Perelygin AA, Zharkikh AA, et al. Characterization of equine and other vertebrate TLR3, TLR7, and TLR8 genes. Immunogenetics 2009;61: 529–39.
9. Gornik K, Moore P, Figueiredo M, et al. Expression of Toll-like receptors 2, 3, 4, 6, 9, and MD-2 in the normal equine cornea, limbus, and conjunctiva. Vet Ophthalmol 2011;14:80–5.
10. Lohmann KL, Vandenplas ML, Barton MH, et al. The equine TLR4/MD-2 complex mediates recognition of lipopolysaccharide from *Rhodobacter sphaeroides* as an agonist. J Endotoxin Res 2007;13(4):235–42.
11. Zhang YW, Davis EG, Blecha F, et al. Molecular cloning and characterization of equine Toll-like receptor 9. Vet Immunol Immunopathol 2008;124:209–19.
12. Quintana AM, Landolt GA, Annis KM, et al. Immunological characterization of the equine airway epithelium and of a primary equine airway epithelial cell culture model. Vet Immunol Immunopathol 2011;140:226–36.
13. Figueiredo MD, Vandenplas ML, Hurley DJ, et al. Differential induction of MyD88- and TRIF-dependent pathways in equine monocytes by Toll-like receptor agonists. Vet Immunol Immunopathol 2009;127:125–34.
14. Kwon S, Gewirtz AT, Hurley DJ, et al. Disparities in TLR5 expression and responsiveness to flagellin in equine neutrophils and mononuclear phagocytes. J Immunol 2011;186:6263–70.
15. Flaminio MJ, Borges AS, Nydam DV, et al. The effect of CpG-ODN on antigen presenting cells of the foal. J Immune based Therap Vacc 2007;5:1.
16. Trent MS, Stead CM, Tran AX, et al. Diversity of endotoxin and its impact on pathogenesis. J Endotoxin Res 2006;12:205–23.
17. Schumann RR. Old and new findings on lipopolysaccharide-binding protein: a soluble pattern-recognition molecule. Biochem Soc Trans 2011;39:989–93.
18. Szatmary Z. Molecular biology of toll-like receptors. Gen Physiol Biophys 2012; 31:357–66.
19. Brikos C, O'Neill LA. Signalling of toll-like receptors. Handb Exp Pharmacol 2008;(183):21–50.
20. Siegemund S, Sauer K. Balancing pro- and anti-inflammatory TLR4 signaling. Nat Immunol 2012;13:1031–3.
21. Aksoy E, Taboubi S, Torres D, et al. The p110δ isoform of the kinase PI(3)K controls the subcellular compartmentalization of TLR4 signaling and protects from endotoxic shock. Nat Immunol 2012;13:1045–54.
22. Darrah PA, Monaco MC, Jain S, et al. Innate immune responses to *Rhodococcus equi*. J Immunol 2004;173:1914–24.
23. Cheevers WP, Archer BG, Crawford TB. Characterization of RNA from equine infectious anemia virus. J Virol 1977;24:489–97.
24. Lambert AJ, Martin DA, Lanciotti RS. Detection of North American Eastern and Western equine encephalitis viruses by nucleic acid amplification assays. J Clin Microbiol 2003;41(1):379–85.
25. Mottahedin A, Paidikondala M, Cholleti H, et al. NF-κB activation by equine arteritis virus is MyD88 dependent and promotes viral replication. Arch Virol 2013;158(3):701–5.
26. Rahman MM, McFadden G. Modulation of NF-kB signaling by microbial pathogens. Nat Rev Microbiol 2011;9:291–306.
27. Wilson JR, de Sessions PF, Leon MA, et al. West Nile virus nonstructural protein 1 inhibits TLR3 signal transduction. J Virol 2008;82(17):8262–71.

28. Liu J, Xu C, Hsu LC, et al. A five-amino-acid motif in the undefined region of the TLR8 ectodomain is required for species-specific ligand recognition. Mol Immunol 2010;47:1083–90.

29. Liu M, Liu T, Bordin A, et al. Activation of foal neutrophils at different ages by CpG oligodeoxynucleotides and *Rhodococcus equi*. Cytokine 2009;48:280–9.

30. Sun WC, Moore JN, Hurley DJ, et al. Effects of stimulation of adenosine A2A receptors on lipopolysaccharide-induced production of reactive oxygen species by equine neutrophils. Am J Vet Res 2007;68:649–56.

31. Biswas SK, Lopez-Collazo E. Endotoxin tolerance: new mechanisms, molecules and clinical significance. Trends Immunol 2009;30:475–87.

32. Kwon S, Vandenplas ML, Figueiredo MD, et al. Differential induction of Toll-like receptor gene expression in equine monocytes activated by Toll-like receptor ligands or TNF-α. Vet Immunol Immunopathol 2010;138:213–7.

33. Walsh C, Gangloff M, Monie T, et al. Elucidation of the MD-2/TLR4 interface required for signaling by lipid IVa. J Immunol 2008;181:1245–54.

34. Bryant CE, Ouellette A, Lohmann K, et al. The cellular Toll-like receptor 4 antagonist E5531 can act as an agonist in horse whole blood. Vet Immunol Immunopathol 2007;116:182–9.

35. Figueiredo MD, Moore JN, Vandenplas ML, et al. Effects of the second-generation synthetic lipid A analogue E5564 on responses to endotoxin in [corrected] equine whole blood and monocytes. Am J Vet Res 2008;69:796–803.

36. Reitschel ET, Cavaillon JM. Richard Pfeiffer and Alexandre Besredka: creators of the concept of endotoxin and anti-endotoxin. Microbes Infect 2003;5:1407–14.

37. Coley WB. The treatment of malignant tumors by repeated inoculations of erysipelas, with a report of ten original cases. Am J Med Sci 1893;105:487–511.

38. Hill AB, Hatswell JM, Topley WW. The inheritance of resistance, demonstrated by the development of a strain of mice resistant to experimental inoculation with a bacterial endotoxin. J Hyg 1940;40:538–47.

39. Burrows GE. Endotoxemia induced by rapid intravenous injection of *Escherichia coli* in anesthetized ponies. Am J Vet Res 1970;31:1967–73.

40. Aggarwal BB, Gupta SC, Kim JH. Historical perspectives on tumor necrosis factor and its superfamily: 25 years later, a golden journey. Blood 2012;119:651–65.

41. MacKay RJ. Association between serum cytotoxicity and selected clinical variables in 240 horses admitted to a veterinary hospital. Am J Vet Res 1992;53(5):748–52.

42. Collatos C, Barton MH, Prasse KW, et al. Intravascular and peritoneal coagulation and fibrinolysis in horses with acute gastrointestinal tract diseases. J Am Vet Med Assoc 1995;207:465–70.

43. Barton MH, Parviainien A, Norton N. Polymyxin B protects horses against induced endotoxemia in vivo. Equine Vet J 2004;36:397–401.

44. Hoshino K, Takeuchi O, Kawai T, et al. Cutting Edge: Toll-like receptor 4 deficient mice are hyporesponsive to lipopolysaccharide: evidence for TLR4 as the LPS gene product. J Immunol 1999;162:3749–52.

45. Lopes MA, Salter CE, Vandenplas ML, et al. Expression of inflammation-associated genes in circulating leukocytes collected from horses with gastrointestinal tract disease. Am J Vet Res 2010;71:915–24.

46. Leise BS, Faleiros RR, Watts M, et al. Laminar inflammatory gene expression in the carbohydrate overload model of equine laminitis. Equine Vet J 2011;43:54–61.

47. Barton MH, Morris DD, Norton N, et al. Hemostatic and fibrinolytic indices in neonatal foals with presumed septicemia. J Vet Intern Med 1998;12:26–35.

48. Steverink P, Sturk A, Rutten V, et al. Endotoxin, interleukin-6 and tumor necrosis factor concentrations in equine acute abdominal disease – relation to clinical outcome. J Endotoxin Res 1995;2:289–99.
49. Senior JM, Proudman CJ, Leuwer M, et al. Plasma endotoxin in horses presented to an equine referral hospital: correlation to selected clinical parameters and outcomes. Equine Vet J 2011;43:585–91.
50. Kane TD, Alexander JW, Johannigman JA. The detection of microbial DNA in the blood: a sensitive method for diagnosing bacteremia and/or bacterial translocation in surgical patients. Ann Surg 1998;227:1–9.
51. Liaudet L, Szabo C, Evgenov OV, et al. Flagellin from gram-negative bacteria is a potent mediator of acute pulmonary inflammation in sepsis. Shock 2003;19: 131–7.
52. Sitaraman SV, Klapproth JM, Moore DA 3rd, et al. Elevated flagellin-specific immunoglobulins in Crohn's disease. Am J Physiol Gastrointest Liver Physiol 2005; 288:G403–6.
53. Lodes MJ, Cong Y, Elson CO, et al. Bacterial flagellin is a dominant antigen in Crohn disease. J Clin Invest 2004;113:1296–306.
54. Sykes BW, Furr MO. Equine endotoxaemia – a state-of-the-art review of therapy. Aust Vet J 2005;83:45–50.
55. Seok J, Warren HS, Cuenca AG, et al. Genomic responses in mouse models poorly mimic human inflammatory diseases. Proc Natl Acad Sci U S A 2013; 110:3507–12.

Ultrasound of the Equine Acute Abdomen

Sarah le Jeune, DVM*, Mary Beth Whitcomb, DVM, MBA

KEYWORDS

- Acute abdomen • Ultrasound • Colic

KEY POINTS

- Ultrasound can be a quick, noninvasive tool in formulating the accurate diagnosis of horses presenting with acute colic, leading to successful treatment and outcome.
- Transcutaneous ultrasound gives immediate information on the volume and type of peritoneal effusion, gastric dilatation and contents; small intestinal contents, motility, wall thickness, and diameter; and large intestinal contents and wall thickness.
- Ultrasound can be useful in distinguishing between strangulating and nonstrangulating small intestinal lesions and can help determine whether a horse should have surgery.
- A low-frequency (2–5 MHz) curvilinear transducer is the transducer of choice for equine transcutaneous abdominal ultrasonography because of its ability to image up to 27 to 30 cm of depth.

INTRODUCTION AND CLINICAL INDICATIONS

Transcutaneous abdominal ultrasonography has become an integral part of the diagnostic workup for the acute abdomen in many equine clinics. A quick and accurate assessment of horses with acute abdominal pain is essential for the formulation of the correct diagnosis, prognosis, and treatment, particularly as it pertains to the initial decision of either medical or surgical management. Abdominal ultrasound is a relatively easy, noninvasive tool to evaluate the anatomic location, wall thickness, motility, and contents of the intestine. Transcutaneous ultrasound is of particular value in patients that cannot undergo rectal palpation due to size (foals or miniature horses), lack of adequate restraint, safe facilities, excessive straining, history of a rectal tear, or where rectal palpation is limited because of advanced pregnancy. Despite limitations caused by the large depth and size of the abdominal cavity of the horse, the presence of osseous ribs encasing the cranial viscera, and varying amounts of gaseous

The authors have nothing to disclose.
Department of Surgical and Radiological Sciences, University of California, 1 Shields Avenue, Davis, CA 95616, USA
* Corresponding author.
E-mail address: sslejeune@ucdavis.edu

Vet Clin Equine 30 (2014) 353–381
http://dx.doi.org/10.1016/j.cveq.2014.04.011
0749-0739/14/$ – see front matter Published by Elsevier Inc.

distension, ultrasound provides valuable information that could not be obtained by other diagnostic methods.[1–3]

Transcutaneous ultrasound examination is a noninvasive method that gives immediate information on the volume and type of peritoneal effusion; gastric dilatation and contents; small intestinal contents, motility, wall thickness, and diameter; and large intestinal contents and wall thickness.[1–7] Ultrasonography has been shown to be a reliable method for the evaluation of normal intestinal wall thickness in horses and ponies[4,8,9] as well as for assessment of strangulating small intestinal lesions[3,6,10–12] and strangulating large colon lesions[10,13,14] as compared with histologic sections.[15]

Originally, the use of abdominal ultrasonography as a diagnostic tool in colic patients was evaluated prospectively in 226 colics.[6] In this study, horses with primary small intestinal lesions had a small intestine (SI) wall thickness of 0.2 to 1.8 cm and a diameter of 3.6 to 13.5 cm without evidence of motility. Horses with peritonitis showed SI motility, wall thickness measurements of 0.5 to 1.3 cm, and diameters of 2 to 5.1 cm. Horses with primary large colon lesions or small colon impactions had ultrasonographic evidence of small intestinal motility, normal SI wall thicknesses, and diameters of 3 to 7.1 cm. More importantly, if distended and amotile SI was detected by ultrasonographic evaluation, the sensitivity, specificity, and positive and negative predictive values for SI strangulation obstructions were 100%. In contrast, detection of abnormal SI via transrectal palpation yielded a sensitivity of only 50%, specificity of 98%, and a positive and negative predictive value of 89% for small intestine strangulation obstructions. This study showed that the use of abdominal ultrasonography in horses with signs of colic is accurate in detecting SI strangulation obstructions.

A recent retrospective study investigated the correlation between abdominal ultrasonographic findings and disease categories that cause abdominal pain requiring surgery in 158 horses.[10] In this study, abdominal ultrasound was performed to assess for free peritoneal fluid, visibility of the left kidney, gastric distention, the appearance and motility of the duodenum, the appearance, motility, and thickness of SI loops, and the appearance and motility of the colon. The most significant findings of this study were that the presence of distended and nonmotile small intestinal loops was associated with strangulating small intestinal obstructions; that increased free peritoneal fluid and distended and thickened SI loops with abnormal motility were associated with a definitive diagnosis involving the SI, that failure to visualize the left kidney was associated with nephrosplenic entrapment, and that thickened large colon was associated with large colon strangulating volvulus. This finding indicates that ultrasound is a useful diagnostic tool to aid in determining whether a horse needs colic surgery.

A protocol for fast, localized abdominal ultrasonography of horses (FLASH) has been recently described.[11] In this protocol, the horse's abdomen is divided into 7 regions (described below under technique) and assessed using alcohol saturation and without clipping. This protocol was evaluated by inexperienced clinicians in 36 horses with colic. In this study, the FLASH examination was completed within approximately 10 minutes and was able to show free peritoneal fluid and abnormal intestinal loops. Thirteen horses were considered surgical colics. Sensitivity, specificity, and positive and negative predictive values for dilated small intestinal loops as an indicator of small intestinal obstruction were similar to that reported by Klohnen and colleagues.[6] These results support the use of the FLASH technique by experienced and inexperienced veterinarians to detect important abdominal abnormalities in equine colic patients.

Technique and Equipment

Although the type of ultrasound machine is often thought to be the most important factor to obtain quality ultrasonographic images, the value of abdominal ultrasound is more heavily influenced by the following factors: patient preparation, individual horse-to-horse variation, availability of ultrasound transducers, technique, experience level of the examiner, and complexity of the abdominal disorder.

Patient preparation
Alcohol saturation is sufficient for imaging the acute abdomen in most instances. In heavily coated or obese horses, clipping the hair with no. 40 blades is often necessary to obtain diagnostic images. Ponies, donkeys, and certain breeds with thick skin and heavy fat deposition, such as Friesians, draft breeds, and Icelandic horses, are notoriously challenging to image and thus often require clipping.

Transducers and ultrasound machines
A low-frequency (2–5 MHz) curvilinear transducer is preferable for abdominal imaging; however, a rectal transducer can provide useful information to aid in the decision-making process for surgical referral. Visibility with a rectal transducer is limited to structures close to the skin surface because of its maximal scanning depth of 10 to 12 cm. Fortunately, abnormal SI is heavy and falls to the dependent portion of the abdomen, usually adjacent to the body wall where it may be detected with a rectal transducer. A rectal transducer can also identify ventral peritoneal fluid accumulations to assist with abdominocentesis. Transrectal ultrasound may be performed with either a traditional linear rectal transducer or a small curvilinear (microconvex) transducer. The latter transducer is quite small and can be readily manipulated within the rectum.

A low-frequency (2–5 MHz) curvilinear transducer is the transducer of choice for equine transcutaneous abdominal ultrasonography because of its ability to image up to 27 to 30 cm of depth. Curvilinear transducers are available for nearly all of today's ultrasound machines and are capable of producing high-quality, diagnostic images in the ambulatory and hospital setting. In addition, the curvilinear arrangement of ultrasound crystals produces a sector-shaped image regardless of scanning depth, resulting in a wider field of view when compared with linear transducers. In contrast, the rectal transducer (a linear transducer) produces a progressively narrower image as the scanning depth is increased.

Scanning technique
Techniques for abdominal ultrasound can roughly be broken down into 3 general categories: the limited examination, the FLASH technique, and the full examination. Variations of these techniques abound, depending on examiner preferences and experience.[4,6,11,16]

Limited examination The limited examination often focuses on the caudoventral abdomen and left caudal intercostal spaces (ICS) in colicking horses. The primary goal is to detect evidence of nephrosplenic entrapment from the renosplenic window and strangulating small intestinal lesions from the ventral abdomen. This examination can be quickly performed in the ambulatory setting to help determine whether surgical referral is indicated. The limited examination is appropriate for beginning and novice abdominal imagers to prevent becoming overwhelmed by the more thorough examinations described below.

FLASH technique The recently described FLASH technique is based in part on FAST (focused assessment with sonography in trauma) techniques used in human emergency clinics.[11] The FLASH technique has been met enthusiastically by practitioners, in part because of its catchy name, but also because it expands beyond the limited examination. The FLASH technique is performed using alcohol saturation in the unclipped horse and divides the horse's abdomen into 7 topographic locations: ventral abdomen, gastric window, splenorenal window, left middle third of the abdomen, duodenal window, right middle third of the abdomen, and thoracic window.

Full examination The full examination divides each side of the abdomen into 3 general regions: (1) paralumbar fossa/flank region from the level of the tuber coxae to the stifle; (2) ICS (5–17th) from the ventral lung margins to costochondral junctions; (3) ventrum from sternum to inguinal region (cranial to caudal) and costochondral junctions to midline (left to right). Each region is thoroughly evaluated in systematic fashion, rather than dividing the abdomen into specific windows as with the FLASH technique. In addition, each ICS is evaluated from the ventral lung margin to the costochondral junctions to ensure imaging of all abdominal structures *and* the ventral thorax to detect pleural/pulmonary abnormalities that can mask as colic. Although this examination can initially seem extensive, it can be performed quickly in colic patients.

Machine settings

Regardless of the technique used, image quality should be optimized by altering frequency settings, time-gain compensation controls, depth settings, and overall gain. Settings will depend on the individual situation. In general, larger horses will require a lower frequency setting for adequate penetration than a foal or young, fit Thoroughbred racehorse, whereby a higher frequency setting of 5 MHz often produces the best image quality. In general, it is best to scan with the highest frequency setting that will result in adequate penetration. Depth settings should be adjusted frequently, depending on the location of the structure of interest. Shallow depth settings (6–12 cm) will give better detail of superficial structures but will not be adequate to visualize deeper abdominal structures. In contrast, scanning with a constant depth setting of 20 to 30 cm will result in subtle findings being overlooked in those structures located close to the skin surface.

Examiner experience and diagnostic complexity

There is little question that ultrasound is highly operator dependent, in both image acquisition and interpretation. Fortunately, the basic questions to be answered with abdominal ultrasound (evidence of strangulating obstructions, nephrosplenic entrapment, peritoneal effusion) in many colicking horses are fairly straightforward. In contrast, less common disorders, such as obstructive cholelithiasis, dissecting aortic root aneurysms, and neoplasia, generally require much more experience to detect and recognize. Findings consistent with colon torsion or right dorsal displacement are more common, but also require more than basic ultrasound skills. In addition, findings such as severe colonic thickening may represent both surgical and medical disorders, colon torsion, or colitis, respectively.[14,17] Interpretation must always consider the clinical picture of the horse, which may not be as straightforward as one might anticipate.

Normal Ultrasonographic Anatomy of the Equine Abdomen

Briefly, the cecum, cecal mesentery, right kidney, right liver lobe, duodenum, and right dorsal colon are evaluated from the right side of the abdomen, and the left kidney, spleen, stomach, and left liver lobe are evaluated from the left side of the horse. The left dorsal colon and ventral colon are seen predominantly in the left ventral abdomen, and the right ventral colon is visualized primarily from the right ventral abdomen. Differentiation between cecum and colon segments is primarily based on location rather than the presence and size of sacculations.[18] Jejunum is most often seen in the ventral abdomen, but may be visible in multiple locations throughout the abdomen.[9]

Left abdomen

The spleen is the predominant feature of the left abdomen, including the ICS and ventrum, and often extends to or slightly to the right of midline (**Fig. 1**). The spleen is homogenously echogenic and should appear hyperechoic to the liver and kidneys. The splenic vein is visible in nearly all horses near the gastrosplenic space. The left kidney is visible deep to the spleen in the left paralumbar fossa region and caudal (15–17th) ICS. The stomach is located dorsal to the spleen and ventral to the lung in the left 10th to 15th ICS. Evaluation is primarily limited to its greater curvature. Gastric contents are not typically visible, unless there are increased luminal fluid contents.[19] The left liver lobe is imaged cranial to the stomach in the left 6th to 10th ICS. The left liver lobe may be situated lateral or medial to the spleen, but should always be hypoechoic to the spleen. Visibility of the left liver lobe is somewhat variable and may not be seen in some horses. Large colon should be visible deep to the spleen. Collapsed to mildly dilated SI loops are often detectable between the spleen and large colon and occasionally in the gastrosplenic space.[9]

Right abdomen

The cecum is visualized from the upper right paralumbar fossa and flank region with its apex extending to the ventral abdomen (**Fig. 2**). The cecal mesentery and lateral cecal artery and vein can be evaluated along this same path,[20] but may not be of particular interest when evaluating the acute abdomen. The right kidney is seen in the caudal

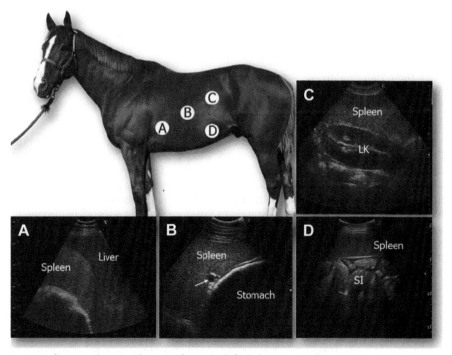

Fig. 1. Reference ultrasound images from the left abdomen. (*A*) The spleen and left liver lobe are seen in the left cranial (6–10th) ICS. (*B*) Gastrosplenic window. The spleen, splenic vein (*arrow*), and stomach are seen in the left mid-ICS. (*C*) Renosplenic window. The left kidney (LK) is seen deep to the spleen in the left paralumbar fossa region and caudal ICS (15–17th). (*D*) SI loops are often identified deep to the spleen in the left caudoventral abdomen.

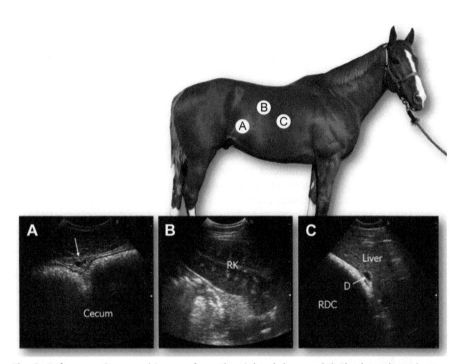

Fig. 2. Reference ultrasound images from the right abdomen: (*A*) The lateral cecal artery and vein are seen within the cecal mesentery (*arrow*). The mesentery can often be followed from this location to the cecal apex. (*B*) The right kidney (RK) is visualized adjacent to the body wall in the right 14th to 17th ICS. (*C*) The right liver lobe is seen ventral to the lung in the right 10th to 15th ICS in many horses. The duodenum (D) and right dorsal colon (RDC) are visible deep to the right liver lobe. The RDC shows a characteristic large radius of curvature.

right ICS (14–17th) adjacent to the body wall. The right liver lobe is visible in the right ICS, usually the 10th to 15th ICS. Margins should be sharp and not extend to or beyond the costochondral junctions. The descending duodenum has a fixed location and is visible in most horses ventral to the right kidney and deep to the right liver lobe in the right 11th to 17th ICS.[9,21] Visibility in the more cranial ICS is highly variable, as the duodenum becomes deeper as it extends to the stomach. The ascending duodenum cannot be visualized with ultrasound. The right dorsal colon is located deep to the right liver lobe in the right ICS and shows a large, smooth radius of curvature. The mixture of luminal feed and gas precludes visualization of the lumen and the far wall of the colon and cecum. Colonic or cecal wall thickness is often difficult to measure in normal horses. The hyperechoic gas/feed contents should not erroneously be included when acquiring wall thickness measurements. Normal colon and cecal wall thickness measurements are somewhat variable between reports, but measurements greater than 3 to 4 mm are generally considered thickened.[8,9,16,18] Interpretation of measurements should consider the degree and distribution of thickening (focal vs diffuse) as well as the detail provided by the image to obtain accurate wall thickness measurements.

Ventrum
The large colon is the dominant feature of the ventral abdomen. Although jejunum can be found in multiple sites throughout the abdomen, common locations for visualization

of small intestinal loops include the inguinal regions, deep to the spleen and occasionally in the gastrosplenic space.[9] SI visibility may be increased in fasted horses.[22] The bladder may be seen caudally in the inguinal region in some horses. Urine may appear variably echoic due to the presence of mucus and crystals. Care should be taken not to confuse a bladder containing echogenic urine for an abdominal abscess. It should be emphasized that evaluation of the entire ventral abdomen is an important part of the ultrasound examination in the acute abdomen, as many abnormalities described in this article are frequently identified in the ventral abdomen.

Gastric Abnormalities

Ultrasonographic evidence of gastric distention in equine colic patients is most often secondary to primary small intestinal lesions and occasionally large intestine disorders (**Fig. 3**). Primary gastric disorders are infrequent and include gastric impaction and gastric neoplasia, such as squamous cell carcinoma (addressed later in this article).[23] In horses with gastric distention due to excess feed or fluid accumulation, the stomach will become visible over a larger number of ICS. Although some authors suggest that gastric visibility over more than 5 ICS is consistent with gastric distention,[16] this is seen routinely during ultrasound examinations in noncolic patients by one author (M.B.W.). Dorsocaudal displacement of the stomach wall is considered ultrasonographic evidence of gastric distention. Due to considerable variability between horses, it is important to obtain a baseline assessment of gastric position to use for comparison during subsequent examinations. This information can then be used to estimate gastric volume and base the need for nasogastric intubation and decompression.[19] Gastric contents are not typically visible in horses with gastric feed impaction, but increased gastric fluid contents may be seen in horses with gastric reflux due to enteritis or other small intestinal disorders. An enlarged radius of curvature may also be noted.

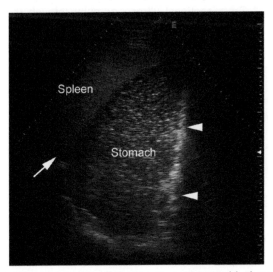

Fig. 3. Ultrasound image of gastric distention in a 31-year-old Thoroughbred gelding admitted for colic due to proximal enteritis. The stomach was visible from the left 8th through 14th ICS and showed an enlarged radius of curvature and a large ventral fluid accumulation with a visible gas-fluid interface (*arrowheads*). Splenic vein (*arrow*). Dorsal is to the right.

Small Intestinal Abnormalities

Abdominal ultrasonography can be very useful in distinguishing between small intestinal distension due to nonsurgical conditions, such as ileus or enteritis, and surgical lesions, such as small intestinal strangulation. Most small intestinal abnormalities and some large intestinal abnormalities create visible small intestinal distention. The increased weight created by the distention causes abnormal loops to migrate to the ventrum (in standing horses) or the dependent portion of the abdomen (in recumbent patients). Small intestinal distension can be seen on transcutaneous ultrasound before being palpated by rectum.[2,24] Small intestinal distension has been defined as a luminal diameter greater than or equal to 5 cm. Increased small intestinal wall thickness is considered greater than or equal to 3 mm.[6,10,12] It should be mentioned that small intestinal distention can also be found in horses with primary large intestine abnormalities.

Small intestinal strangulating obstructions

As mentioned previously, visualization of distended and amotile loops of SI is highly associated with small intestinal strangulating lesions (**Fig. 4**).[2,10,12] Careful evaluation of the ventral abdomen is important in all patients because strangulated loops tend to fall to the dependent portion of the abdomen. Affected loops are often round in shape, as opposed to compressed or triangular in shape, as can be seen in horses with enteritis or ileus. The presence of both distended and collapsed small intestinal loops can also be seen. Wall thickness measurements can be normal or increased, sometimes in the same horse, especially when imaging the strangulated portion of bowel (thickened) rather than the dilated loops proximal to the obstruction (nonthickened) (**Fig. 5**).

Intussusception

Small intestinal intussusceptions can occasionally be diagnosed in foals and rarely in adult horses.[25,26] Cross-sectional ultrasonography through the intussusception often reveals a typical bull's-eye or target appearance (**Fig. 6**).[25] Abdominal

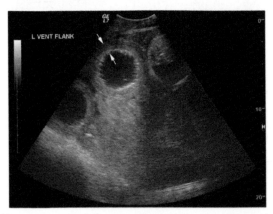

Fig. 4. Ultrasound image from the left ventral flank region showing marked small intestinal thickening and distention (*arrows*) in a 2-year-old Warmblood gelding with small intestinal volvulus found at surgery. Although wall thickness is not shown, a measurement of 1 to 1.5 cm can be extrapolated from the depth scale on the right side of the image. (*Courtesy of* Dr Erin Byrne, Alamo Pintado Equine Medical Center, Los Olivos, CA.)

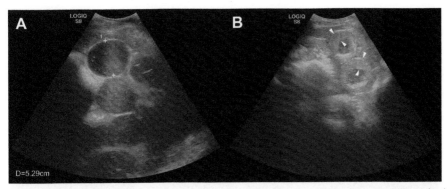

Fig. 5. Ultrasound images from an adult horse with a strangulating lipoma. (*A*) Marked small intestinal distention is noted (luminal diameter = 5.29 cm). (*B*) In the same horse, severe SI wall thickening of up to 1.5 cm (*arrowheads*) is also evident, which likely represents the strangulated portion of bowel. Twenty-seven feet of jejunum were resected at surgery. (*Courtesy of* Dr Erin Byrne, Alamo Pintado Equine Medical Center, Los Olivos, CA.)

ultrasonography in foals may improve the recognition of these surgical lesions and improve the potential for successful treatment. Similar to most small intestinal lesions, small intestinal intussusceptions are typically edematous and fluid-filled and fall to the most dependent portion of the abdomen, which should be a consideration when performing ultrasound on a recumbent foal.

Proximal enteritis

Horses with ileus due to enteritis show varying degrees of small intestinal and gastric distention (**Fig. 7**). Small intestinal motility is reduced but usually not absent; however, affected horses with large numbers of turgid and amotile small intestinal loops have been reported.[11] In such cases, differentiation between surgical and nonsurgical lesions can be challenging. A positive response to repeated decompression via

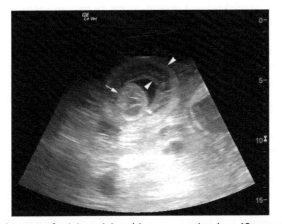

Fig. 6. Ultrasound image of a jejuno-jejunal intussusception in a 12-year-old Arab gelding with a 36-hour history of colic. This image was obtained from the ventral abdomen and shows the characteristic bull's-eye appearance created by the intussusceptum (*arrows*) within the severely thickened intussuscipiens (*arrowheads*).

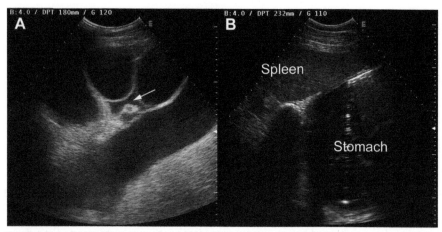

Fig. 7. Ultrasound images from a horse with proximal enteritis. (*A*) Prominently dilated and hypomotile small intestinal loops are seen throughout the ventral abdomen. Pockets of anechoic peritoneal fluid (*arrow*) are also visible. (*B*) Gastric distention due to increased fluid contents was present in this horse and is a common feature of proximal enteritis. Both findings can also be seen in horses with strangulating lesions, making differentiation between conditions challenging.

nasogastric intubation may point to a diagnosis of proximal enteritis. Wall thickness may be thickened or normal in affected horses.

Other small intestinal lesions

Small intestinal thickening is not an uncommon finding in colic patients with other non-strangulating small intestinal lesions. Possible diagnoses include inflammatory bowel disease (IBD), hypertrophy due to distal obstruction, and less commonly, idiopathic muscular hypertrophy or neoplasia (addressed later in this article). All may present with a previous history of colic episodes. Differentiation between conditions is challenging, especially in the emergency setting, unless a mass or abscess is also found in conjunction with SI thickening. Luminal, mural, or extramural masses can all cause proximal distention and mural thickening. Thickening may involve all layers or only the muscular layer. Horses with idiopathic muscular hypertrophy show severe thickening that is limited to the muscularis layer of the SI (**Fig. 8**A).[27,28] Horses with IBD may show segmental or diffuse SI thickening (see **Fig. 8**B). Some IBD horses may also show cecal lymphadenopathy; however, this finding is not pathognomonic for this condition.[20] Diagnosis may rely on a positive response to corticosteroids in nonsurgical cases or via surgical biopsy/resection.

Duodenal abnormalities

Although duodenal abnormalities are uncommon primary causes of colic, the duodenum should be evaluated for distention, thickening, or alterations in motility. Visualization of the normal duodenum may not be practical in the emergency setting, because it may be collapsed and visibility may require waiting for peristalsis. In horses with enteritis or other jejunal disorders, the duodenum may appear persistently or intermittently distended and hypomotile.[10,11] Severe distention should prompt closer evaluation for a duodenal mass or other obstruction (**Fig. 9**A). Severe duodenal thickening has been seen in foals and horses with duodenitis and duodenal ulceration. Duodenoscopy may be beneficial in such cases (see **Fig. 9**B).

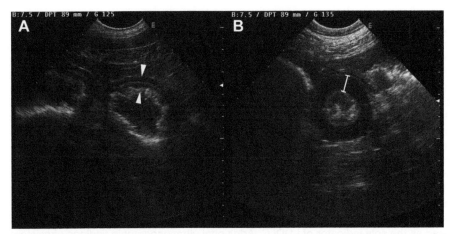

Fig. 8. Ultrasound images of severe small intestinal thickening from 2 different horses. (*A*) Severe diffuse thickening involving all SI layers (*arrowheads*) in a horse with recurrent colic bouts due to IBD, later diagnosed as eosinophilic-lymphoplasmacytic enterocolitis. (*B*) Severe thickening of the muscularis layer (*bracket*) in an adult miniature horse due to idiopathic muscular hypertrophy. Mucosal and submucosal thickening are also present. Approximately 15 feet of affected SI were resected at surgery, after which the colic bouts resolved.

Large Intestinal Abnormalities

Left dorsal displacement

Left dorsal displacement of the large colon (LDDLC) or nephrosplenic entrapment of the large colon is a cause of acute colic in horses, particularly in large Warmblood breeds. Even though the colon can be palpated by rectum as it courses laterally to the spleen into the nephrosplenic space, transcutaneous ultrasound can be used to confirm the diagnosis. LDDLC is typically diagnosed ultrasonographically when a

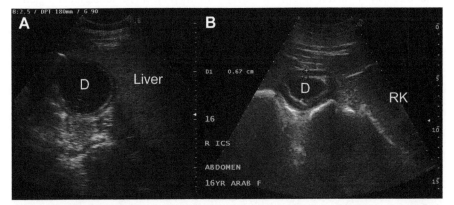

Fig. 9. Ultrasound images of the descending duodenum (D) from 2 different horses with colic. Images were obtained from the right 15th and 16th ICS, respectively. Dorsal is to the right. (*A*) Duodenal distention and hypomotility are present in this 23-year-old Morgan gelding diagnosed with splenic B-cell lymphoma at necropsy. A definitive reason for the duodenal findings was not identified. (*B*) Moderate duodenal thickening (6.7 mm) is seen in this 16-year-old Arab mare with multiple recurrent episodes of colic. Diffuse thickening was also noted of small intestinal loops throughout the ventral abdomen. RK, right kidney.

gas echo is identified dorsal to the spleen and obliterating the dorsal splenic border and left kidney, or when the colon is observed laterally to the spleen (**Fig. 10**). In the original study investigating the use of ultrasound to diagnose and to monitor the nonsurgical correction of LDDLC, ultrasound was found to be a very reliable aid in the diagnosis of LDDLC and in confirming correction of the displacement after a nonsurgical rolling procedure.[29] Ultrasound has since been integrated into standard practice in the management of this condition.[30,31] In the original report, no false positives and few false negatives were identified, indicating a high specificity with a lower sensitivity to diagnose LDDLC with ultrasound.[29] It is the authors' experience that unaffected horses, horses with other displacements of the large colon, and even large colon torsions can potentially have a similar appearance on ultrasound, particularly in obliterating the left kidney. This obliteration has been reported in other studies, including one where only 2 of 7 horses without a visible left kidney were found to have LDDLC and another study that reported 18 of 143 false positive examinations.[10,11] Therefore, nonvisualization of the left kidney on ultrasound should not be used as the sole indicator of LDDLC. Additional ultrasonographic findings consistent with LDDLC include splenic enlargement and ventral displacement, often extending past the ventral midline.

Right dorsal displacement

Ultrasonographic findings associated with right dorsal displacement include dilated mesenteric vessels on the right side of the abdomen, reported as near the costochondral junctions in 1 to 2 ICS.[32,33] In the authors' experience, abnormally distended vessels are most often found in the right 10th to 12th ICS and are oriented *parallel* with the ribs.[34] This nearly vertical orientation is almost perpendicular to the horizontal orientation of the large colon and its mesenteric vasculature in the normal horse (**Fig. 11**). Although surgical intervention is recommended in such cases, it is interesting that some horses without a surgical option have resolved with only supportive treatment. It is important not to confuse this finding with the normal appearance of the lateral cecal artery and vein. Cecal vessels are oriented somewhat vertically but are located further caudally in the abdomen, extending from the paralumbar fossa/flank region to the ventral abdomen.

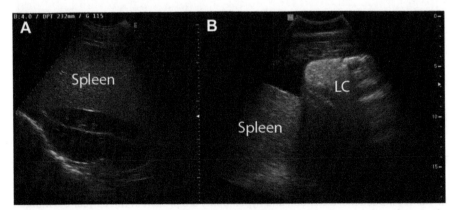

Fig. 10. (*A*) Normal renosplenic window. The left kidney is visible deep to the spleen in the caudal ICS. (*B*) In this horse with nephrosplenic entrapment, the left kidney is obscured by large colon (LC), which has migrated lateral and dorsal to the spleen. Peritoneal effusion is also present in this image. Dorsal is to the right in both images.

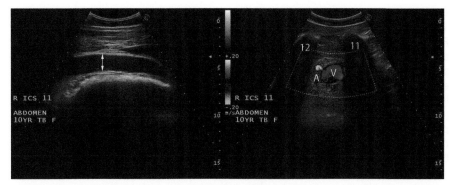

Fig. 11. Longitudinal (*left*) and transverse (*right*) ultrasound images of a severely distended mesenteric vein (*double headed arrows*, V) in a horse with right dorsal displacement. Both images were obtained from the right 11th ICS with the transducer oriented parallel to the ribs in the left image and perpendicular to ribs 11 and 12 in the right image. Venous blood flow was visible with both B-mode and color Doppler imaging. The smaller artery (A) is visible adjacent to the dilated vein on the transverse image.

Colon torsion

Large colon torsion is a common cause of severe colic in horses and ultrasound is typically not essential in establishing the correct diagnosis and treatment plan. However, in atypical cases where the colon is not completely strangulated and pain is not severe, ultrasound can be a useful diagnostic tool for this condition. Abutarbush[13] described a technique wherein the identification of nonsacculated large colon in the left ventral portion of the abdomen indicated a large colon volvulus, and the degree and location of the volvulus could be accurately estimated by ultrasound.[13] In a prospective study conducted by Pease and colleagues,[14] a colon wall thickness greater than or equal to 9 mm accurately predicted strangulating large colon torsion (**Fig. 12**) with a 100% specificity and 67% sensitivity using a ventral abdominal window.

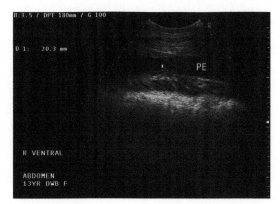

Fig. 12. Severe colonic thickening in a 13-year-old broodmare that presented for tachycardia (up to 120 bpm) and lying down at 4 days postpartum. Although this image was obtained from the right ventral abdomen, similar thickening was present throughout the right abdomen and left ventral abdomen. Peritoneal effusion (PE) is also visible. A 360° colon torsion was found and corrected at surgery.

Colitis

The term colitis may apply to multiple conditions that cause colonic inflammation. Right dorsal colitis is a common concern among equine veterinarians, and its clinical and ultrasonographic features have been described in multiple reports.[35–37] The ultrasound focus of these reports was on the right dorsal colon; however, colonic thickening consistent with colitis can be found throughout the colon in affected horses.[17] In the authors' experience, thickening is infrequently isolated to the right dorsal colon (**Fig. 13**). As such, examination should extend beyond the right dorsal colon in all suspect cases to more fully document the extent of involvement. Horses with acute infectious or inflammatory colitis may demonstrate similar ultrasonographic findings. Differentiation often relies on patient history and other clinical features.

Intussusception

Intussusceptions involving the large intestine include cecocecal, cecocolic, colocolic, ileocecal, and ileocecocolic intussusceptions. Ultrasound findings include a target sign similar to that seen with small intestinal intussusceptions, but because of their larger size, luminal fluid can be seen within the concentric rings of the intussusception.[38–40] Preoperative differentiation of the specific anatomic structures involved is challenging in large intestinal intussusceptions. In some horses, a masslike appearance may be present, especially if scanning immediately adjacent to the intussusception.[34] A closer look will often reveal the presence of an intussusceptum and intussuscepiens (**Fig. 14**). Because most large colon intussusceptions involve the cecum, identification requires imaging on the right side of the abdomen, including the right flank, paralumbar fossa, and ICS, regions that tend to be less frequently evaluated in colic patients. In one study of cecal intussusceptions, ultrasound was used to diagnose 3 of 37 ileocecal intussusceptions, 3 of 5 cecocecal intussusceptions, and 12 of 19 cecocolic intussusceptions; however, ultrasound was not performed in all cases.[41] These findings are similar to other studies on large intestinal intussusceptions where ultrasound was used to diagnose only 2 of 30 cases[42] and 2 of 8 cases,[43]

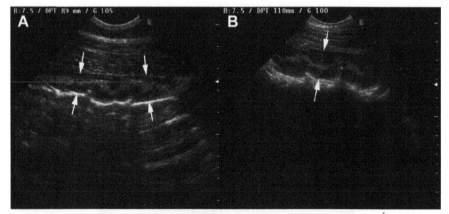

Fig. 13. Severe colonic thickening in a 15-year-old Thoroughbred mare with colic. (*A*) The right dorsal colon is severely thickened and shows an edematous, layered appearance (*arrows*). (*B*) Severe colonic thickening (*arrows*) was also seen throughout the abdomen, including the cranioventral abdomen as shown in this image. Wall thickness measurements ranged from 9.4 to 15 mm and involved nearly all visible portions of the colon. The horse recovered with conservative treatment.

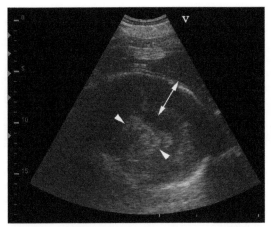

Fig. 14. Ultrasound image of a colocolic intussusception in a 17-year-old Tennessee Walker mare with a 2-week history of mild colic. The inner intussusceptum is seen (*arrowheads*) within the severely thickened and edematous outer intussuscipiens (*double headed arrow*). The intussusception was visible from the right 11th to 13th ICS. Surgical reduction was unsuccessful, and the horse was euthanized after the owner declined large colon resection.

respectively. Admittedly, both studies included years wherein the use of abdominal ultrasound was not yet embraced in colic patients.

Sand/Enteroliths

Sand accumulations within the large colon and enterolithiasis are typically diagnosed with abdominal radiographs as they cannot be imaged adequately with ultrasound. However, a Finnish group investigated the correlation of radiographic with ultrasonographic findings (large intestinal motility and localization relative to the ventral abdominal wall) in horses with sand accumulations.[44] In that study, the specificity of ultrasonography in detecting ventrally located sand accumulations was 87.5% and the sensitivity was 87.5%, but small and more dorsally located accumulations were difficult to detect. The authors were able to identify ultrasonographically the ventral aspect of sand accumulations as a hyperechoic line, allowing for an estimation of the length of the accumulation, but not the height, and the large intestine had decreased or absent motility. A weakness of the study was the lack of blinding of the ultrasonographers to the radiographic findings; it is the authors' experience that sand accumulations are not reliably identified on ultrasound.

Peritoneal Fluid

Ultrasound is helpful to determine the location of peritoneal fluid for abdominocentesis and to assess the quantity and character of fluid in horses with peritoneal effusions. Peritoneal fluid is not typically visible, but a few small pockets of anechoic fluid may be found in normal horses.[9] Although the ventral abdomen is the most common location to visualize peritoneal fluid, it is not unusual to detect fluid dorsal to the spleen in the gastrosplenic window and dorsal to the spleen and left kidney in the left caudal ICS (renosplenic window) in some horses (**Fig. 15**). Visualization of fluid in the latter location should not be overinterpreted as evidence of severe effusion based solely on its dorsal location. Although significant effusion may be present, this location is merely a potential space for small effusions to accumulate. Assessment of quantity is

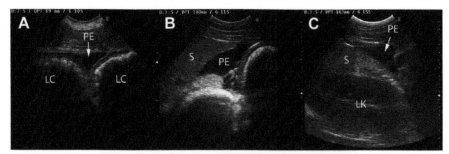

Fig. 15. Common locations to visualize peritoneal effusion (PE) in the equine abdomen. (*A*) Ventral abdomen. A small pocket of anechoic effusion is visible in this horse with mild to moderate large colon (LC) thickening. (*B*) Gastrosplenic window. Peritoneal fluid may be detected dorsal to the spleen (S) in horses with mild to moderate peritoneal effusion. (*C*) Renosplenic window. Effusion may also be visible dorsal to the spleen (S) and left kidney (LK) in the left caudal ICS.

somewhat subjective, but multiple small- to moderate-size pockets of peritoneal effusion throughout the abdomen is generally considered abnormal.

A rectal transducer is often sufficient to detect ventral fluid accumulations, depending on the size and body condition of the horse. In thin or young horses, 4 to 8 cm of scanning depth may be adequate. Horses with a thick retroperitoneal fat layer will require an increased scanning depth, which may exceed the capabilities of a rectal transducer. Most horses have some retroperitoneal fat. Fat should not be mistaken for peritoneal fluid or liver, which can occur in difficult to image horses due to the hypoechoic and somewhat speckled appearance of fat (**Fig. 16**). Close inspection will reveal that fat will indent on peristalsis of overlying bowel. Swirling will be noted in horses with cellular effusion.

The character of peritoneal fluid should be also be evaluated, especially when faced with large effusions. Hemorrhagic fluid generally shows a fairly homogeneous and cellular appearance. It characteristically shows swirling with gentle external ballottement, respiratory, or peristaltic movements (**Fig. 17**). Ultrasound should then be

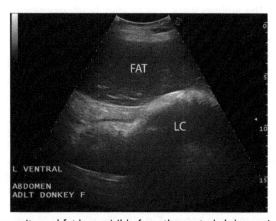

Fig. 16. Thick retroperitoneal fat layer visible from the ventral abdomen in an adult donkey. Retroperitoneal fat of varying thicknesses is visible throughout the ventral abdomen in nearly all horses/equids. Its hypoechoic and speckled appearance should not be confused with hepatic parenchyma or cellular peritoneal effusion. LC, large colon.

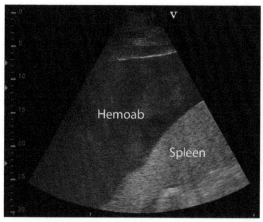

Fig. 17. Severe cellular-appearing effusion in a horse with hemoabdomen (Hemoab) due to splenic fracture (not visible in this image). Note the somewhat homogeneous appearance of the fluid, which swirls with movement of the GI tract and shifting of the horse's weight.

directed to identify the source of the hemoperitoneum, which may include splenic hematoma or fracture, hemangiosarcoma, and other neoplasias.[45–47] Fluid that is heterogeneous, contains debris, or contains hyperechoic gas echoes is most consistent with bowel rupture. Severe anechoic effusion may be due to uroabdomen (**Fig. 18**) or neoplasia such as metastatic peritoneal carcinomatosis or mesothelioma. Uroabdomen is an uncommon cause of acute colic and is more likely in foals secondary to urinary bladder rupture. However, it can be found in adult horses with urinary rupture due to urolithiasis and should be suspected when large amounts of anechoic fluid are present within the abdominal cavity even if a urine-distended bladder can be seen, because the urine leakage can result from other parts of the urinary tract.

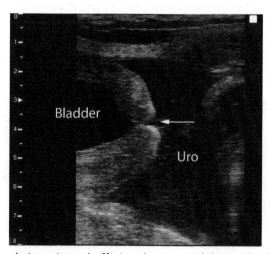

Fig. 18. Severe anechoic peritoneal effusion due to uroabdomen (Uro) in a 12-year-old Quarter Horse mare with bladder rupture (*arrow*) considered to be traumatic in origin. Although the bladder wall defect is visible in this case, it may not be identified in all cases. The tear was surgically repaired, and the mare recovered uneventfully.

Masses, Neoplasia, and Abscessation

Although horses with abdominal abscessation or neoplasia more commonly exhibit clinical signs, such as fever of unknown origin, weight loss, or chronic intermittent colic, they can present with acute colic signs especially if the mass is causing gastro-intestinal (GI) obstruction.[48–56] Masses and abscesses can be found throughout the abdomen, but large masses are often found on the ventral abdomen due to their dependent nature.[55] Diagnosis usually requires a low-frequency curvilinear transducer and a skilled eye. Masses palpable by rectum can be evaluated with a linear rectal transducer; however, transrectal examination with a small curvilinear transducer (microconvex) may provide a more complete evaluation due to its wider, sector-shaped image. Transcutaneous ultrasound is often necessary to completely evaluate masses palpable by rectum due to scanning depth limitations of rectal and microcon-vex transducers.

Abdominal neoplasia

The most common intestinal tumors are lymphoma and adenocarcinoma.[56] Small intestinal lymphoma tends to produce annular thickening of the intestinal wall. Affected loops are often visible on the dependent abdominal floor (**Fig. 19**). Differen-tials for annular thickening include idiopathic muscular hypertrophy,[27,28] IBD,[57] and muscular hypertrophy due to a distal obstruction. A trial with corticosteroids may help to differentiate between neoplasia and IBD. Cecal lymphadenopathy may be found in horses with intestinal neoplasia (see **Fig. 19B**), but may also be present in horses with infectious or inflammatory conditions.[20] In contrast to lymphoma, adeno-carcinoma tends to produce focal or solitary masses (**Fig. 20**), although diffuse colonic infiltration has been seen by the authors. Proximal small intestinal distention ± mural thickening may be evident due to functional obstruction. Gastrointestinal stromal cell tumors are less common and tend to produce solitary masses with or without proximal small intestinal distention and mural thickening (**Fig. 21**). Tumors often involve the cecum. Interestingly, affected horses may be asymptomatic.[49,52] Leiomyomas and leiomyosarcomas have also been described.[56]

Additional tumor types that can cause clinical signs of colic include large granulosa cell tumors (**Fig. 22**), splenic lymphoma (**Fig. 23**), and gastric squamous cell carci-noma, among others. Gastroscopy is typically the imaging modality of choice for the diagnosis of gastric squamous cell carcinoma, but ultrasound can detect proliferative masses emanating from the gastric wall in the gastrosplenic space in some horses.[23]

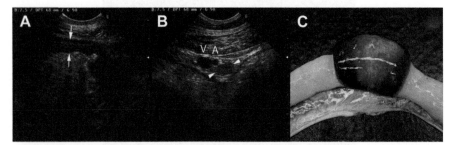

Fig. 19. Small intestinal lymphoma in a 23-year-old Quarter Horse mare. (*A*) Severe small intestinal thickening (*arrows*) was present throughout the ventral abdomen. (*B*) Enlarged cecal lymph nodes (*arrowheads*) were seen adjacent to the lateral cecal artery (A) and vein (V) in the right paralumbar fossa region. (*C*) Postmortem specimen of the same horse showing severe annular small intestinal thickening due to T-cell lymphoma.

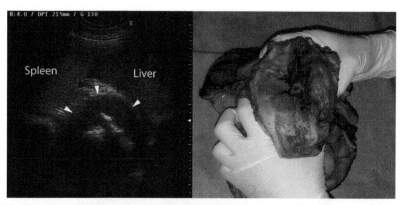

Fig. 20. Ultrasound image and corresponding surgical specimen from a horse with adeno-carcinoma involving the large colon. Severe thickening (2–3 cm) of the large colon wall (*arrowheads*) and an irregular lumen was visible deep to the left liver lobe and spleen from the left 5th through 7th ICS. The owner opted for exploratory celiotomy, and the mass was removed via colon resection.

Abdominal abscessation

The classic appearance for abscessation is a spherical structure containing echogenic fluid contents and a well-defined capsule. This appearance is more often seen with mesenteric abscesses due to *Streptococcus zooepidemicus* or *Streptococcus equi* subspecies *equi*.[54] Although *Rhodococcus equi* abscesses can create a similar appearance (**Fig. 24**), poorly marginated abscesses of mixed echogenicity were re-ported in a study of 11 foals with intra-abdominal abscessation.[55] Abscessation due to *Corynebacterium pseudotuberculosis* typically involves abdominal organs (liver, kidneys, and spleen, in that order). Mesenteric abscesses due to this pathogen are relatively rare, and colic is uncommon.[58]

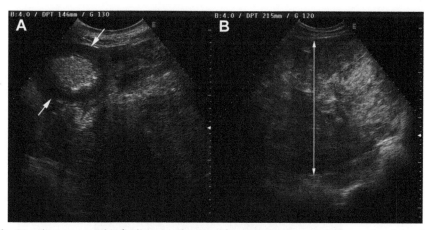

Fig. 21. Ultrasonographic findings in a horse with a large GI stromal cell tumor involving the cecum. (*A*) Severe annular small intestinal thickening involving the muscular layer (*arrows*) was detected near the large solitary mass (*B, double headed arrow*). Both were visualized from the right paralumbar fossa and inguinal region in a 21-year-old Arab gelding with mild colic, inappetence, and weight loss. The mass measured 16 cm × 19 cm × 16 cm. The horse was euthanized 2 weeks later due to declining condition. Necropsy confirmed GI stro-mal cell tumor.

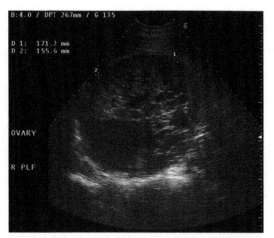

Fig. 22. Large granulosa cell tumor (15.6 cm × 17.1 cm) of the right ovary visible from the right paralumbar fossa/flank region. This granulosa cell tumor was only partially visible and palpable via transrectal ultrasound. Transcutaneous ultrasound allowed assessment of its full size to aid in surgical planning.

Abdominal abscesses may also show irregular margins with heterogeneous, solid-appearing contents that may appear similar to masses or neoplasia. Ultrasonographic differentiation between neoplasia and abscessation is not straightforward in such cases. Anaerobic abscesses typically show an additional component of hyperechoic gas echoes (**Fig. 25**). This finding should prompt abdominal radiographs to rule out a migrating metallic foreign body such as a wire. Ultrasound can be used to monitor response to treatment in horses with abscessation.[58] Ultrasound-guided aspiration is generally not recommended for mesenteric abscesses due to the risk for bowel

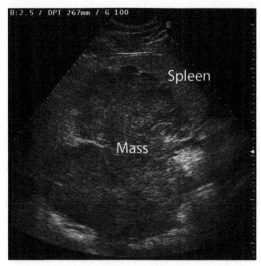

Fig. 23. Large heterogeneous splenic mass in a 4-year-old Thoroughbred racehorse with recent colic. The heterogeneous, cauliflower-like appearance of this mass is highly suggestive of splenic lymphoma. Ultrasound-guided biopsy confirmed the diagnosis.

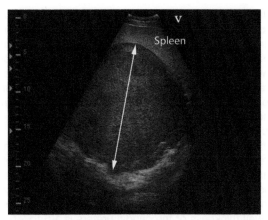

Fig. 24. Large mesenteric abscess (*double headed arrow*) due to *R equi* in a 3-month-old Thoroughbred foal. A well-defined capsule is apparent in this case, but poorly defined abscesses of mixed echogenicity may also be found. The abscess extended for a length of 28 cm along the ventral abdomen.

perforation or leakage but has been used successfully for the diagnosis of hepatic, renal, and splenic abscesses due to *C pseudotuberculosis*.[58]

Other

Urolithiasis

Horses with obstructive urolithiasis may present with signs of colic, but more often show hematuria and azotemia.[59–61] In horses with urinary obstruction due to uretero-liths or cystoliths, distention of the renal pelvis may be the only finding on

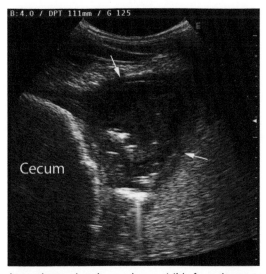

Fig. 25. Anaerobic abscess (*arrows*) at the cecal apex visible from the ventral abdomen. Hyper-echoic gas echoes within the abscess raised the suspicion for a migrating foreign body, which was later confirmed on abdominal radiographs. The abscess was surgically resected via partial typhlectomy. Partial splenectomy was also necessary due to adhesions to the spleen.

transcutaneous ultrasound. Palpation of a bladder stone may be found during rectal palpation of colic patients and should be confirmed via transrectal ultrasound (**Fig. 26**); the entire urinary tract should be scanned to rule out additional uroliths. This scan is especially important in horses with ureteral obstruction as the primary cause of colic, in which case removal of the bladder stone will not resolve the horse's clinical signs. Ultrasound is also important to evaluate for significant underlying renal disease to aid in prognostication. It is important to perform ultrasound before cystoscopy to prevent the introduction of gas that would obscure ultrasonographic visualization of urinary structures.

Uroliths, regardless of their location, appear as hyperechoic structures that cast hard shadows. Ureteroliths can be found along the length of the ureter via transrectal ultrasonography and are often associated with distention and ureteral thickening proximal to the obstructing stone (**Fig. 27**A). The left and right ureters are evaluated individually by starting at the bladder trigone and following each as far cranially as possible. Normal wall thickness of the caudal ureters is 1.5 to 2.0 mm, with motility used to differentiate between ureters and deferent ducts/ampulla in male horses.[62] Cystoliths located at the trigone region may also create ureteral thickening and distention, and even renal pelvic distention in some cases.

Nephroliths are recognized as hyperechoic structures within the renal pelvis that cast hard shadows. Renal sludge appears similarly but may produce a "dirty" or less distinct shadow (see **Fig. 27**B). Differentiation between nephroliths and renal sludge is not straightforward. Care should be taken not to misinterpret the hyperechoic appearance of the renal pelvis as nephrolithiasis.

Cholelithiasis

Hepatic causes of colic primarily include obstructive cholelithiasis[63–65]; however, this is an uncommon finding in the authors' experience. In contrast to that seen with urolithiasis, hepatoliths can be of variable echogenicity and can create variable acoustic

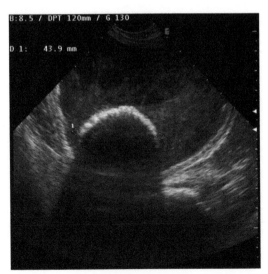

Fig. 26. Cystolith in a 17-year-old Argentinian sport horse gelding with frequent posturing to urinate. Ultrasound of the urinary tract revealed no additional uroliths or renal or ureteral abnormalities. The cystolith was removed under general anesthesia. Five years later, the horse has had no recurrence of urolithiasis.

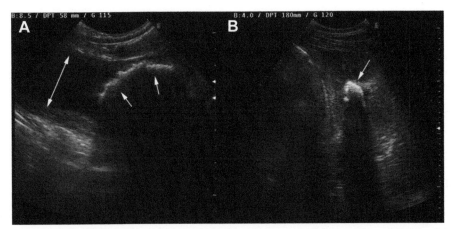

Fig. 27. Ultrasound images from a 4-year-old Warmblood gelding with urolithiasis. (*A*) Transrectal ultrasound shows a large ureterolith (*small arrows*) within the right ureter and severe ureteral distention (*double headed arrow*) proximal to the stone. (*B*) Transcutaneous ultrasound reveals one of several nephroliths (*arrow*) within the right renal pelvis. Note the characteristic strong shadow cast by the stone. Additional findings included bilateral renal enlargement, thickened renal cortices, and changes consistent with chronic renal failure. The horse was euthanized due to poor prognosis based on the extent and severity of ultrasonographic findings throughout the urinary tract.

shadowing (**Fig. 28**A).[65] Biliary distention is a concurrent finding in most cases, seen as a "parallel channel sign" whereby the bile duct becomes distended adjacent to portal veins (see **Fig. 28**B). In some cases, hepatoliths cannot be visualized if located deep within the biliary tree. Additional findings that may be confused with hepatoliths include hepatic granulomas,[66] biliary fibrosis, or biliary inflammation. These findings can create distal shadowing, and when diffuse, a starry sky pattern has been described in a group of horses with hepatic granulomas.[66] Hepatoliths should be differentiated by their location within the biliary tree.

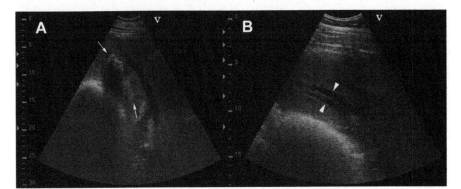

Fig. 28. Ultrasound images from a 14-year-old Thoroughbred breeding stallion with colic and icterus. (*A*) Hyperechoic hepatoliths (*arrows*) are seen within the biliary tree of the left liver lobe. These stones cast variably dirty shadows, in contrast to that seen with uroliths. (*B*) No hepatoliths were seen at any location within the right liver lobe; however, a parallel channel sign (*arrowheads*) is evident secondary to distention of the bile ducts adjacent to the portal vein.

Thoracic and cardiac causes of colic

Pleuritis Horses with pleurodynia caused by pleuritis may occasionally present with acute colic signs **(Fig. 29)**. It is therefore recommended to evaluate the ventral lung margins during abdominal ultrasound, which will aid in the detection of comet tails and/or pleural effusion that may implicate the thoracic cavity as the source of clinical signs. A few small comet tails are generally considered clinically insignificant, especially in older horses that may have residual scarring from previous lung infections. Diffuse or large comet tails, pulmonary consolidation, or pleural effusion should prompt complete thoracic examination.

Pericarditis Although relatively uncommon, pericardial effusion with or without cardiac tamponade and tachycardia may produce clinical signs consistent with acute colic **(Fig. 30)**. Pleural effusion can appear similar to pericardial effusion in some horses. Identification of fluid that extends around the apex of the heart is often seen in horses with large pericardial effusions.

Aortic root disease Aortic root aneurysms and aortocardiac fistulas are rare painful conditions that frequently present as colic patients.[67,68] Mature breeding stallions are most often affected, but aortic root disease has been reported in mares and geldings. Aortic root disease should be considered in horses with severe tachycardia unresponsive to sedation, a continuous right-sided murmur, electrocardiographic evidence of ventricular tachycardia (usually monomorphic), and lack of significant GI signs on colic examination. Echocardiographic diagnosis can be challenging for the novice imager, and definitive diagnosis may require a specialist familiar with echocardiography. Ultrasound findings include dilatation of the aortic root, fistula formation that extends into the right atrium or right ventricle, and/or dissecting tracts through the interventricular septum **(Fig. 31)**. Prognosis is poor. Reported survival times range from a few days to 12 months in most cases. Sudden death has been reported.

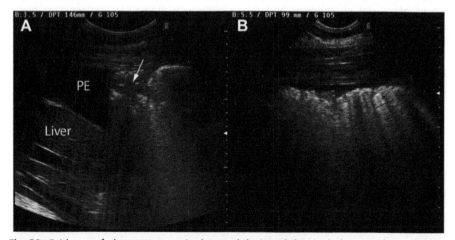

Fig. 29. Evidence of pleuropneumonia detected during abdominal ultrasound in a 14-year-old Quarter Horse gelding presenting for colic and occasional grunting. (*A*) Moderate pleural effusion (PE) and ventral pulmonary consolidation (*arrow*) were evident within the cranioventral thorax bilaterally. (*B*) Multiple diffuse comet tails were detected throughout the right ventral lung fields. The lung was adhered to the parietal pleural surface at this location (right 11–12th ICS) and showed jerky movements with respiration. The horse was treated for primary pleuropneumonia and recovered uneventfully.

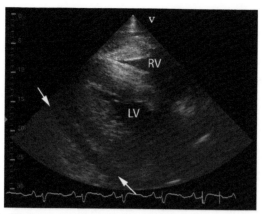

Fig. 30. Pericardial effusion (*arrows*) in a horse presenting for colic. No abdominal abnormalities were detected. Echocardiography was performed due to persistent tachycardia and an irregular rhythm. Toxin screens were negative. Effusive-constrictive pericarditis due to an unknown toxin was suspected. The horse responded to supportive care. LV, left ventricle; RV, right ventricle.

Diaphragmatic hernia Diaphragmatic hernia can cause acute colic in adults and foals.[69,70] Preoperative diagnosis can be difficult because of the absence of affected intestine within the abdominal cavity and the lack of peritoneal fluid changes. Depending on the size of the defect within the diaphragm, either small or large intestine can herniate. Typically, large defects result in large intestinal herniation that leads to dyspnea and respiratory distress. In contrast, small defects more often result in small intestinal herniation and strangulating obstruction that lead to acute colic signs. Ultrasonography of the thorax and cranial abdomen can allow visualization of intestinal contents within the thorax even when pleural effusion is present (**Fig. 32**). Diagnosis is not always straightforward, especially in cases with large colon herniation,

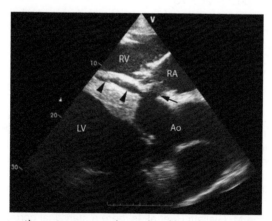

Fig. 31. Dissecting aortic root aneurysm (*arrowheads*) and aortocardiac fistula (*arrow*) extending into the right atrium in a 27-year-old thoroughbred breeding stallion that presented for tachycardia and a continuous right-sided murmur after collapsing immediately following breeding. The dissecting tract extended 8 to 9 cm into the interventricular septum. Ao, aorta; LV, left ventricle; RA, right atrium; RV, right ventricle. (*Courtesy of* Johanna Reimer, DVM, DACVIM, Lexington, KY.)

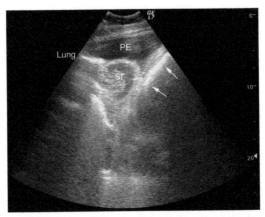

Fig. 32. Ultrasound image from a 17-year-old Quarter Horse gelding with a diaphragmatic hernia involving 10 feet of SI. A SI loop is seen within the pleural space between the lung and diaphragm (*arrows*). Pleural effusion (PE) is also seen. Dorsal is to the left. (*Courtesy of* Dr Erin Byrne, Alamo Pintado Equine Medical Center, Los Olivos, CA.)

where the hyperechoic bowel wall may appear similar to lung. Even horses with small intestinal herniation may require close scrutiny to appreciate the presence of amotile bowel within the pleural space.

REFERENCES

1. Fischer AT Jr. Advances in diagnostic techniques for horses with colic. Vet Clin North Am Equine Pract 1997;13(2):203–19.
2. Scharner D, Rotting A, Gerlach K, et al. Ultrasonography of the abdomen in the horse with colic. Clin Tech Equin Pract 2002;1:118–24.
3. Freeman S. Ultrasonography of the equine abdomen: findings in the colic patient. In Pract 2002;24:262–73.
4. Freeman S. Ultrasonography of the equine abdomen: techniques and normal findings. In Pract 2002;24:204–11.
5. Henry Barton M. Understanding abdominal ultrasonography in horses: which way is up? Compend Contin Educ Vet 2011;33(9):E2.
6. Klohnen A, Vachon AM, Fischer AT Jr. Use of diagnostic ultrasonography in horses with signs of acute abdominal pain. J Am Vet Med Assoc 1996;209(9): 1597–601.
7. Fontaine GL, Hanson RR, Rodgerson DH, et al. Ultrasound evaluation of equine gastrointestinal disorders. Compend Cont Educ Pract Vet 1999;21:253–62.
8. Bithell S, Habershon-Butcher JL, Bowen IM, et al. Repeatability and reproducibility of transabdominal ultrasonographic intestinal wall thickness measurements in thoroughbred horses. Vet Radiol Ultrasound 2010;51(6):647–51.
9. Epstein K, Short D, Parente E, et al. Gastrointestinal ultrasonography in normal adult ponies. Vet Radiol Ultrasound 2008;49(3):282–6.
10. Beccati F, Pepe M, Gialletti R, et al. Is there a statistical correlation between ultrasonographic findings and definitive diagnosis in horses with acute abdominal pain? Equine Vet J Suppl 2011;(39):98–105.
11. Busoni V, De Busscher V, Lopez D, et al. Evaluation of a protocol for fast localised abdominal sonography of horses (FLASH) admitted for colic. Vet J 2011; 188(1):77–82.

12. Porzuczek A, Kielbowicz Z, Haines G. The use of percutaneous abdominal ultrasound examination in diagnosing equine small intestinal disorders. Pol J Vet Sci 2012;15(4):759–66.
13. Abutarbush SM. Use of ultrasonography to diagnose large colon volvulus in horses. J Am Vet Med Assoc 2006;228(3):409–13.
14. Pease AP, Scrivani PV, Erb HN, et al. Accuracy of increased large-intestine wall thickness during ultrasonography for diagnosing large-colon torsion in 42 horses. Vet Radiol Ultrasound 2004;45(3):220–4.
15. Freeman SL, Mason PJ, Staley C. Comparison of ultrasonographic and histological assessment of normal and strangulated intestine in the horse. Eur J Ultrasound 2001;13:1–35.
16. Reef VB. Adult abdominal ultrasonography. In: Reef VB, editor. Equine diagnostic ultrasound. Philadelphia: WM Saunders Co; 1998. p. 273–363.
17. Biscoe EW, Whitcomb MB, Vaughan B, et al. Ultrasonographic features and clinical outcome in horses with severe large colon thickening: (2003-10). Am Assoc Equine Pract 2011;57:459.
18. Hendrickson EH, Malone ED, Sage AM. Identification of normal parameters for ultrasonographic examination of the equine large colon and cecum. Can Vet J 2007;48(3):289–91.
19. Lores M, Stryhn H, McDuffee L, et al. Transcutaneous ultrasonographic evaluation of gastric distension with fluid in horses. Am J Vet Res 2007;68(2):153–7.
20. Vaughan B, Whitcomb MB, Pusterla N. Ultrasonographic findings in 42 horses with cecal lymphadenoapthy. Am Assoc Equine Pract 2013;59:238.
21. Kirberger RM, van den Berg JS, Gottschalk RD, et al. Duodenal ultrasonography in the normal adult horse. Vet Radiol Ultrasound 1995;36(1):50–6.
22. Mitchell CF, Malone ED, Sage AM, et al. Evaluation of gastrointestinal activity patterns in healthy horses using B mode and Doppler ultrasonography. Can Vet J 2005;46(2):134–40.
23. Taylor SD, Haldorson GJ, Vaughan B, et al. Gastric neoplasia in horses. J Vet Intern Med 2009;23(5):1097–102.
24. Cavalleri JM, Bienert-Zeit A, Feige K. Examination of horses with acute colic - clinical pathology and diagnostic imaging. Tierarztl Prax Ausg G Grosstiere Nutztiere 2013;41(2):124–34 [quiz: 135] [in German].
25. Bernard WV, Reef VB, Reimer JM, et al. Ultrasonographic diagnosis of small-intestinal intussusception in three foals. J Am Vet Med Assoc 1989;194(3):395–7.
26. Fontaine-Rodgerson G, Rodgerson DH. Diagnosis of small intestinal intussuception by transabdominal ultrasonography in 2 adult horses. Can Vet J 2001;42(5):378–80.
27. Chaffin MK, Fuenteabla IC, Schumacher J, et al. Idiopathic muscular hypertrophy of the equine small intestine: 11 cases (1980-1991). Equine Vet J 1992;24(5):372–8.
28. Dechant JE, Whitcomb MB, Magdesian KG. Ultrasonographic diagnosis-idiopathic muscular hypertrophy of the small intestine in a miniature horse. Vet Radiol Ultrasound 2008;49(3):300–2.
29. Santschi EM, Slone DE Jr, Frank WM 2nd. Use of ultrasound in horses for diagnosis of left dorsal displacement of the large colon and monitoring its nonsurgical correction. Vet Surg 1993;22(4):281–4.
30. van Harreveld PD, Gaughan EM, Valentino LW. A retrospective analysis of left dorsal displacement of the large colon treated with phenylephrine hydrochloride and exercise in 12 horses (1996-98). N Z Vet J 1999;47(3):109–11.

31. Abutarbush SM, Naylor JM. Comparison of surgical versus medical treatment of nephrosplenic entrapment of the large colon in horses: 19 cases (1992-2002). J Am Vet Med Assoc 2005;227(4):603–5.

32. Grenager NS, Durham MG. Ultrasonographic evidence of colonic mesenteric vessels as an indicator of right dorsal displacement of the large colon in 13 horses. Equine Vet J Suppl 2011;(39):153–5.

33. Ness SL, Bain FT, Zantingh AJ, et al. Ultrasonographic visualization of colonic mesenteric vasculature as an indicator of large colon right dorsal displacement or 180 degrees volvulus (or both) in horses. Can Vet J 2012;53(4):378–82.

34. Whitcomb MB. Advanced abdominal ultrasound for chronic colic. In: American College of Veterinary Surgeons: the surgical summit. San Diego (CA): 2005. p. 39–44.

35. Cohen ND. Right dorsal colitis. Equine Vet Educ 2002;14:212–9.

36. Cohen ND, et al. Medical management of right dorsal colitis in 5 horses: a retrospective study (1987-1993). J Vet Intern Med 1995;9(4):272–6.

37. Jones SL, Davis J, Rowlingson K. Ultrasonographic findings in horses with right dorsal colitis: five cases (2000-2001). J Am Vet Med Assoc 2003;222(9):1248–51.

38. Taintor J, Stewart AJ, Christmann U, et al. What is your diagnosis? Cecocolic intussusception. J Am Vet Med Assoc 2004;225(12):1829–30.

39. Valdes-Martinez A, Waguespack RW. What is your diagnosis? Cecocolic intussusception. J Am Vet Med Assoc 2006;228(6):847–8.

40. Lores M, Ortenburger AI. Use of cecal bypass via side-to-side ileocolic anastomosis without ileal transection for treatment of cecocolic intussusception in three horses. J Am Vet Med Assoc 2008;232(4):574–7.

41. Bell RJ, Textor JA. Caecal intussusceptions in horses: a New Zealand perspective. Aust Vet J 2010;88(7):272–6.

42. Martin BB Jr, Freeman DE, Ross MW, et al. Cecocolic and cecocecal intussusception in horses: 30 cases (1976-1996). J Am Vet Med Assoc 1999;214(1):80–4.

43. Boussauw BH, Domingo R, Wilderjans H, et al. Treatment of irreducible caecocolic intussusception in horses by jejuno(ileo)colostomy. Vet Rec 2001;149(1):16–8.

44. Korolainen R, Ruohoniemi M. Reliability of ultrasonography compared to radiography in revealing intestinal sand accumulations in horses. Equine Vet J 2002;34(5):499–504.

45. Conwell RC, Hillyer MH, Mair TS, et al. Haemoperitoneum in horses: a retrospective review of 54 cases. Vet Rec 2010;167(14):514–8.

46. Dechant JE, Nieto JE, Le Jeune SS. Hemoperitoneum in horses: 67 cases (1989-2004). J Am Vet Med Assoc 2006;229(2):253–8.

47. Pusterla N, Fecteau ME, Madigan JE, et al. Acute hemoperitoneum in horses: a review of 19 cases (1992-2003). J Vet Intern Med 2005;19(3):344–7.

48. Arnold CE, Chaffin MK. Abdominal abscesses in adult horses: 61 cases (1993-2008). J Am Vet Med Assoc 2012;241(12):1659–65.

49. Del Piero F, Summers BA, Cummings JF, et al. Gastrointestinal stromal tumors in equids. Vet Pathol 2001;38(6):689–97.

50. East LM, Savage CJ. Abdominal neoplasia (excluding urogenital tract). Vet Clin North Am Equine Pract 1998;14(3):475–93, v–vi.

51. Elce YA. Infections in the equine abdomen and pelvis: perirectal abscesses, umbilical infections, and peritonitis. Vet Clin North Am Equine Pract 2006;22(2):419–36, ix.

52. Hafner S, Harmon BG, King T. Gastrointestinal stromal tumors of the equine cecum. Vet Pathol 2001;38(2):242–6.
53. Magee AA, Ragle CA, Hines MT, et al. Anorectal lymphadenopathy causing colic, perirectal abscesses, or both in five young horses. J Am Vet Med Assoc 1997;210(6):804–7.
54. Pusterla N, Whitcomb MB, Wilson WD. Internal abdominal abscesses caused by Streptococcus equi subspecies equi in 10 horses in California between 1989 and 2004. Vet Rec 2007;160(17):589–92.
55. Reuss SM, Chaffin MK, Schmitz DG, et al. Sonographic characteristics of intra-abdominal abscessation and lymphadenopathy attributable to Rhodococcus equi infections in foals. Vet Radiol Ultrasound 2011;52(4):462–5.
56. Taylor SD, Pusterla N, Vaughan B, et al. Intestinal neoplasia in horses. J Vet Intern Med 2006;20(6):1429–36.
57. Scott EA, Heidel JR, Snyder SP, et al. Inflammatory bowel disease in horses: 11 cases (1988-1998). J Am Vet Med Assoc 1999;214(10):1527–30.
58. Pratt SM, Spier SJ, Carroll SP, et al. Evaluation of clinical characteristics, diagnostic test results, and outcome in horses with internal infection caused by Corynebacterium pseudotuberculosis: 30 cases (1995-2003). J Am Vet Med Assoc 2005;227(3):441–8.
59. Ehnen SJ, Divers TJ, Gillette D, et al. Obstructive nephrolithiasis and ureterolithiasis associated with chronic renal failure in horses: eight cases (1981-1987). J Am Vet Med Assoc 1990;197(2):249–53.
60. Schott HC. Hematuria. In: Robinson NE, editor. Current therapy in equine medicine. Philadelphia: W. B. Saunders Company; 1997. p. 489–91.
61. Schumacher J, Schumacher J, Schmitz D. Macroscopic hematuria of horses. Equine Vet Educ 2002;14(4):201–10.
62. Diaz OS, Smith G, Reef VB. Ultrasonographic appearance of the lower urinary tract in fifteen normal horses. Vet Radiol Ultrasound 2007;48(6):560–4.
63. Johnston JK, Divers TJ, Reef VB, et al. Cholelithiasis in horses: ten cases (1982-1986). J Am Vet Med Assoc 1989;194(3):405–9.
64. Peek SF, Divers TJ. Medical treatment of cholangiohepatitis and cholelithiasis in mature horses: 9 cases (1991-1998). Equine Vet J 2000;32(4):301–6.
65. Reef VB, Johnston JK, Divers TJ, et al. Ultrasonographic findings in horses with cholelithiasis: eight cases (1985-1987). J Am Vet Med Assoc 1990;196(11):1836–40.
66. Carlson KL, Chaffin MK, Corapi WV, et al. Starry sky hepatic ultrasonographic pattern in horses. Vet Radiol Ultrasound 2011;52(5):568–72.
67. Marr CM, Reef VB, Brazil TJ, et al. Aorto-cardiac fistulas in seven horses. Vet Radiol Ultrasound 1998;39(1):22–31.
68. Sleeper MM, Durando MM, Miller M, et al. Aortic root disease in four horses. J Am Vet Med Assoc 2001;219(4):491–6, 459.
69. Santschi EM, Juzwiak JS, Moll HD, et al. Diaphragmatic hernia repair in three young horses. Vet Surg 1997;26(3):242–5.
70. Firth EC. Diaphragmatic hernia in horses. Cornell Vet 1976;66(3):353–61.

Evaluation of the Colic in Horses: Decision for Referral

Vanessa L. Cook, VetMB, PhD[a], Diana M. Hassel, DVM, PhD[b],*

KEYWORDS

- Horse • Colic • Diagnostic tests • Evaluation

KEY POINTS

- A thorough evaluation of the horse with colic allows early identification of cases that need referral for intensive medical or surgical intervention.
- Early referral improves the horse's prognosis and reduces client cost by allowing intervention while the horse is systemically stable.
- Evaluation should start with a detailed history, thorough physical examination, rectal examination, and passage of a nasogastric tube.
- More advanced diagnostics, including transabdominal ultrasonography, abdominocentesis, and point-of-care measurement of lactate and glucose, can aid in the decision for referral.

INTRODUCTION: NATURE OF THE PROBLEM

Colic is the most common emergency in equine practice with approximately 4 out of every 100 horses having an episode of colic each year.[1] Of the horses that are evaluated by a veterinarian in private practice, approximately 7% to 10% have a lesion that requires surgical correction.[2] Although this may be obvious with severe, acute strangulating obstructions, most colic cases are not quite as black and white. Early identification and referral of horses with a surgical lesion is critical to obtain a successful outcome. Early referral allows general anesthesia and surgery to occur while the horse is systemically stable and intestinal damage is mild, and this decreases postoperative morbidity and mortality and reduces client cost. Many owners would consider taking their horse to a referral hospital for evaluation of colic, and with the excellent success in treatment of geriatric horses with colic,[3] age should not be considered a negative factor in the decision to refer.

The authors have nothing to disclose.
[a] Department of Large Animal Clinical Sciences, Michigan State University College of Veterinary Medicine, 736 Wilson Road, East Lansing, MI 48824, USA; [b] Department of Clinical Sciences, College of Veterinary Medicine & Biological Sciences, Colorado State University, 300 West Drake Road, Fort Collins, CO 80523, USA
* Corresponding author.
E-mail address: dhassel@colostate.edu

Vet Clin Equine 30 (2014) 383–398
http://dx.doi.org/10.1016/j.cveq.2014.04.001
0749-0739/14/$ – see front matter © 2014 Elsevier Inc. All rights reserved.

The veterinary practitioner should thoroughly assess the horse on the first visit and appropriately analyze the findings and offer treatment options. This analysis includes obtaining the signalment of the patient, a thorough history, a complete physical examination including transrectal palpation and nasogastric intubation, and performance of appropriate diagnostic tests and procedures. Accumulation of this information will provide the tools to dictate whether referral to a center with surgical capabilities is appropriate. Referral is necessary not only for surgical intervention but also for advanced intensive medical management such as 24-hour monitoring, antiendotoxic therapies, advanced fluid therapy administration, trocarization, or for a second opinion before euthanasia.

PATIENT HISTORY AND SIGNALMENT

Although patient history in itself does not indicate the need for referral, a thorough history and consideration of patient signalment can provide key information toward identifying the specific cause of colic. This knowledge could lead to a more expedited referral in horses with surgical conditions and likely an improved outcome.

Use of a standardized colic history form is recommended to ensure important historical information is not omitted and to streamline the history-taking process. Important components of the history that should be included are the following:

- Duration, nature of onset, and severity of colic signs
- Current diet and recent dietary changes
- Appetite, water intake, and access to water
- Fecal and urine output and consistency
- Reproductive status
- Whether the horse has had prior colic episodes
- History of diarrhea, laminitis, or other medical conditions
- Medications administered
- Vaccination and deworming status and protocol
- Dental care
- Prior surgeries
- Presence of sand or dirt access
- Primary use of the horse
- Current housing and recent changes in management
- Whether other horses on the property have clinical signs of illness
- Whether the horse is a cribber or windsucker
- Locations the horse has lived and recent travel history

There are several specific historical findings that may lead the clinician to consider particular diagnoses. The characteristic signs the patient has demonstrated are one of the most useful components of the history to assist with diagnosis. Did the patient display acute, severe signs initially? If the onset of colic was not observed, is there physical evidence of severe signs of colic such as skin abrasions over prominent points over the head or hips (**Fig. 1**)? This acute onset of severe pain most commonly is associated with a strangulating obstruction. Once the intestine becomes devitalized, the signs of pain may also abate to some degree, making the determination of the need for surgery more difficult. Stoic, aged horses presenting this way with strangulating small intestinal obstructions may be misdiagnosed with duodenitis/proximal jejunitis until progression of disease ensues. Delays in surgical treatment may lead to a poorer prognosis from advanced systemic disease resulting from the presence of necrotic bowel.

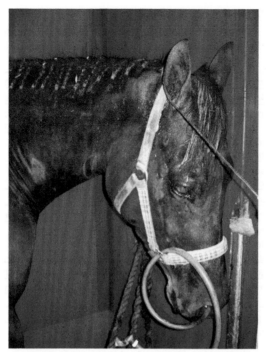

Fig. 1. Horse showing evidence of severe prior colic with abrasions over prominent points on the head.

Another component of the history that is useful in decision making is noting what medications have previously been administered by the owner or trainer. Consider the presence of these medications when observing the horse's degree of pain as it is likely the presence of drugs such as flunixin meglumine will attenuate the clinical signs.

Table 1 contains historical variables that may be associated with particular diagnoses and that may have an impact on the decision for surgery.

Signalment of the patient (age, breed, and sex) can also provide important clues to what type of process should be on the differential list of the clinician. A list of differential diagnoses that should be taken into account based on specifics of patient signalment is provided in **Table 2**.

Horses at increased risk for a surgical condition based on history, signalment, and physical examination findings should be transported to a facility with surgical capabilities at the earliest possible time point.

PHYSICAL EXAMINATION

The basic physical examination, when combined with signalment and history, will often provide the information needed to determine whether surgery is needed in a given colic case. Key components of the physical examination for the colic include

- Pain assessment and general appearance
- Heart rate
- Temperature
- Respiratory rate

Table 1
Patient historical variables that may be associated with particular diagnoses and may aid in the decision for early referral

Historical Variable	Diagnosis Association
Acute onset, severe colic	Strangulating obstruction
Insidious onset colic of several days duration	Nonstrangulating obstruction/displacement
History of recurrent colic episodes	Sand colic; enterolithiasis; gastric or colonic ulcers; impaction; gas colic
Limited access to water/absent or concentrated urine output	Large colon impaction
Feces: diarrhea observed early on followed by progressive colic[35]	Small colon impaction
Feces: persistent soft or watery feces	Colitis
Dull mentation and inappetance	Colitis; non-GI origin systemic diseases
Variable pain followed by signs of shock (sweating, muscle fasciculations and reluctance to move)[4]	GI rupture
Mild to moderate colic followed by severe colic	Secondary LC displacement or LC volvulus
Colic minimally/unresponsive to alpha-2 agonists	Strangulating obstruction
Changes in feed type or quantity of consumption[36,37]:	
Feeding of coastal Bermuda grass hay (East coast)	Ileal impaction
Change to lower-quality fibrous feed	Colon or cecal impaction
Increase in feeding of concentrates	Proximal enteritis[38] or large colon displacement/volvulus from gas production
Alfalfa hay as predominant forage source[39]	Enterolithiasis
Access to moldy hay or grain	Proximal enteritis/gastritis/enterocolitis
History of gradual weight loss and intermittent soft stool	Sand impaction
Feeding on the ground or access to sandy soil	Sand impaction
Recent anthelmintic administration in a young horse[40]	Ascarid impaction
History of chronic NSAID use for musculoskeletal problems[41]	Right dorsal colitis/gastric ulceration
Geographic location—current or recent:	
California	Enterolithiasis
Arizona, Florida, or regions with sandy soils	Sand colic
UK, Northern Mainland Europe, or South America[42]	Equine grass sickness
History of prior colic surgery	Recurrence of original problem/adhesions

Abbreviations: GI, gastrointestinal; NSAID, nonsteroidal antiinflammatory drug.

- Auscultation of gastrointestinal motility
- Perfusion indices (mucous membrane color and capillary refill, jugular refill, extremity temperature)
- Hydration indices (mucous membrane moisture, skin turgor)
- Palpation of digital pulses (pulse strength and temperature of lower limb/hoof)

Table 2
Differential diagnoses to be considered relative to patient signalment

Signalment	Differential Diagnoses
Age: neonate (0–30 d)	Meconium impaction (0–2 d); clostridial enteritis/enterocolitis; strangulating obstruction (small intestinal [SI] volvulus, scrotal hernia); atresias
Age: <2 y of age	Foreign body obstruction[43]; ascarid impaction[44]; intussusception[45]
Age: aged (>12 y)	SI strangulating lipoma; fecalith or large colon impaction
Breed: Arabian/Morgan	Enterolithiasis[39]
Breed: American miniature	Fecalith[46]; sand impaction; enterolithiasis[39,46,47]
Breed: Standardbred/Andalusian draft	Inguinal hernia (stallions)[48–50]
Sex: stallion	Inguinal hernia[49]
Sex: mare—pregnant	Uterine torsion; uterine artery rupture (peri-partum)[51]
Sex: mare—post-partum	Colonic volvulus; uterine artery rupture; mesenteric hematoma/rent

- Rectal palpation
- Passage of nasogastric tube for detection of gastric reflux

Key components of the physical examination to be discussed in greater detail that play strong roles in the decision for surgery include pain assessment with general appearance, heart rate, temperature, gastrointestinal motility, rectal palpation, and presence of gastric reflux.

Pain Assessment and General Appearance

General appearance assessment should include pain assessment, degree of abdominal distension, stance, and body condition scoring. As described earlier in patient history, physical evidence of a prior severe painful episode or observed severe uncontrolled pain is often associated with a strangulating obstruction. A "shocky" or "depressed" appearance following an episode of colic along with reluctance to walk is often associated with intestinal rupture[4] or is observed in stoic horses with strangulating lesions of the small intestine. Degree of abdominal distension has been shown to be an effective discriminating variable for medical versus surgical management of colic.[5] Similarly, the need to administer more than one analgesic treatment to control pain has been associated with the need for surgery.[6] When a specific diagnosis has not been made, lack of response to analgesic administration or resumption of colic after analgesic administration should be considered as a need for surgery.[6] Body condition evaluation may also provide clues as to underlying cause of the colic episode. Horses with sand accumulation tend to have lower body condition scores,[7] and horses with enterolithiasis on an alfalfa-rich diet tend to have higher body condition scores. A poor body condition may also indicate underlying disease processes, inadequate nutrition, or poor dentition.

Heart Rate

Elevation in heart rate, along with other abnormalities in cardiovascular parameters, has been found to be predictive of mortality in several studies evaluating prognosis in colic.[8–10] However, caution should be used in relying on heart rate alone to predict outcome, particularly in horses with normal heart rates, because wide variations exist in between individuals in tolerance to pain and a normal heart rate may exist in the presence of severe gastrointestinal disease. When combined with other physical examination parameters, elevation in heart rate is a useful tool for judging the severity of a disease process because it often indicates severe pain or circulatory compromise. Horses with colic combined with cardiovascular compromise and hypovolemia need aggressive treatment and should have ready access to a referral center. Signs of hypovolemia include tachycardia heart rate (HR>60), cool extremities, delayed jugular refill, variable mucous membrane color, delayed capillary refill time (>2 sec), and diminished peripheral pulse quality.

Temperature

It is important to obtain the body temperature in a horse with colic because this may provide insight into the underlying cause. An exception to this would be the violent, uncontrolled colic that is clearly in need of surgical exploration. Because pneumorectum will often result in a falsely low temperature, body temperature should always be obtained before performing a rectal palpation. Rectal temperature is most often normal or subnormal in the surgical colic case. Subnormal temperatures may be associated with cardiovascular compromise. It is rare to perform surgery for colic on a febrile horse. Exceptions to this may be septic peritonitis and some horses with sand impaction may have low-grade fevers likely as a consequence of chronic mucosal inflammation and bacterial translocation. Although many sand impactions may be treated successfully medically, concurrent colonic displacement often dictates the need for surgical intervention. Horses with concurrent signs of colic with a fever often have an inflammatory or infectious condition such as colitis or duodenitis/proximal jejunitis (DPJ). Similarly, horses with internal abscesses and concurrent peritonitis may be febrile and show signs of colic if adhesions of bowel to the abscess result in gastrointestinal obstruction. In general, be wary of surgical intervention of the febrile horse until further diagnostic tests can help elucidate the underlying cause.

Gastrointestinal Motility

Gastrointestinal motility may be increased in horses with spasmodic colic or phases of colitis and these most often may be managed effectively with medical therapy. Decreased or absent borborygmi is more commonly associated with mechanical obstruction (strangulating or nonstrangulating) or conditions resulting in the systemic inflammatory response syndrome and may be exacerbated by dehydration, electrolyte imbalances, or cardiovascular compromise. Horses with decreased or absent borborygmi have significantly increased odds of requiring surgery compared with horses with normal intestinal sounds.[6] If a horse with colic is demonstrating evidence of progressive intestinal motility as evidenced by both auscultation and passage of feces, surgical intervention is often not required.

Rectal Palpation

The rectal examination is the most useful diagnostic component of the physical examination because, in experienced hands, it can often provide a diagnosis and the degree of distention of bowel can readily be recognized. Commonly diagnosed conditions identified during transrectal palpation include nephrosplenic entrapment (left dorsal displacement of the colon), right dorsal displacement of the colon, cecal impaction, pelvic flexure impaction, colonic volvulus, inguinal herniation, small colon impaction, abdominal masses, gastrointestinal rupture, and detection of small intestinal distention. Serial rectal palpation, particularly in a colicky horse that has minimal abnormalities on its first rectal palpation, is an essential means of assessing progression of disease and the need for surgical intervention.

A systematic approach to transrectal palpation is recommended, ensuring that adequate restraint has been applied. Horses that object to palpation should be restrained with the combination of an alpha2-agonist (xylazine hydrochloride) and an opioid (butorphanol). If straining is present, use of low-dose N-butylscopolammonium bromide (NBB; Buscopan, Boehringer Ingelhiem Vetmedica Inc, St Joseph, Mo.) (0.1–0.15 mg/kg) and use of topical lidocaine in the rectum can be helpful in both improving reach to palpable structures and reducing the risk for iatrogenic rectal tears. The use of NBB will result in an increase in heart rate for up to an hour[11] and will substantially change the way the bowel feels. What once felt moderately to severely gas distended may feel much more compressible and less severely distended when NBB is administered.

Key features to assess for when performing rectal palpation include evidence of any form of distension or displacement along with the location (cecum, large colon, small colon, or small intestine) and type (gas, fluid, or impaction) of distension. Presence of edema within the wall of the palpated intestine should also be noted. Rectal examination findings that often indicate the need for surgical intervention include distention of the small intestine, distended and displaced large colon, severe distention or impaction of any viscus that cannot be resolved with medical therapy, or presence of a palpable foreign body. Older horses with wounds that indicate a severe episode of colic (see **Fig. 1**) with a palpable impaction often have strangulating small intestinal disease. Differentiating between a "dehydrated colon" and a true colonic impaction is essential in these cases. True colonic impactions tend to be "taut" or distended with an absence of undulations from colonic haustra on the surface of the bowel and will typically be larger in diameter than a colon containing dry, firm, dehydrated ingesta from lack of fluid content from the small intestine.

The ability to routinely identify normal visceral anatomy, including the descending colon containing fecal balls, the large colon and pelvic flexure, the caudal border of the spleen, the left kidney, the nephrosplenic ligament, the vertically oriented ventral band of the cecum, the urinary bladder, and the female reproductive tract, will prove useful when abnormalities are present. For example, when the ventral band of the cecum is displaced medially and the ventral colon with its characteristic taenia (bands) and haustra (sacculations) is palpable to the right of the ventral band of the cecum, a right dorsal displacement is present. Ultrasonographic examination of the right lateral body wall can confirm these rectal palpation findings.

Presence of Gastric Reflux

Passage of a nasogastric tube is an essential component of a colic examination, particularly in horses showing signs of severe abdominal pain. A key feature of an overly distended stomach is the inability to pass a nasogastric tube through the cardiac sphincter into the stomach. Access to the stomach is most critical in these cases, yet can be very difficult. Confirmation that an enlarged stomach is present is made by visualizing the stomach extending beyond the 13th intercostal space on ultrasound examination of the left lateral abdomen. Methods that may be used to facilitate passage of the tube include small volume fluid infusion while applying constant pressure and lidocaine infusion into the tube or administration of NBB (Buscopan) to promote relaxation of the cardia.

Once a tube has successfully been passed into the stomach, the nature of the gastric content can provide important clues toward cause of the disease. Large volumes of gastric reflux (>4 L) often indicate a more severe disease process, and referral should be considered. An increased pH of the gastric secretions (>5) is suggestive of a small intestinal origin to the fluid accumulation, whereas orange to red color with a strong foul odor may be associated with some form of proximal enteritis (DPJ). Wide variations exist in appearance of reflux with DPJ. DPJ can result in large volumes of gastric reflux and may create a diagnostic dilemma. It is difficult to differentiate DPJ from strangulating or nonstrangulating small intestinal obstructions in some cases. It is important to try to differentiate DPJ from other surgical small intestinal diseases, because prognosis is likely to be affected if delays in surgical intervention occur with strangulating diseases of the small intestine. Surgical intervention for treatment of DPJ is contraindicated however because it is associated with decreased survival and increased complications.[12] A thorough discussion of history in combination with adjunctive diagnostics including a complete blood count, abdominal ultrasound, and an enzyme-linked immunosorbent assay for *Clostridium difficile* toxins on gastric reflux may provide the necessary clues to help differentiate DPJ from other forms of small intestinal obstruction.

In summary, physical examination findings that often indicate the need for referral and surgical intervention include one or more of the following:

- Severe abdominal discomfort requiring repeated analgesic administration
- Gross and progressive abdominal distention
- Tachycardia (HR>60) and/or signs of hypovolemia
- Absence of auscultable intestinal motility
- Abnormal rectal palpation findings: severe progressive distention of a viscus; displaced large colon; distended small intestine; edematous walls of the large colon; extremely firm or extensive impactions of the large colon, small colon, or ileum; or a palpable foreign body, enterolith or fecalith.
- Gastric reflux volume exceeding 4 L

Caution should be exercised when considering surgery in horses with an absence of abdominal pain or distension, an elevated body temperature greater than 102°F, or significant abnormalities in their blood consistent with an inflammatory intestinal condition (marked leukocytosis or neutropenia).

IMAGING AND ADDITIONAL TESTING

Additional diagnostic tests can provide information that may guide the veterinarian in determining if referral is required. However, none of these tests should be considered in isolation. Instead, the entire evaluation, including a through physical examination, should be considered when making the decision for referral.

Transabdominal Ultrasound

Transabdominal ultrasound has revolutionized the veterinarian's ability to detect gastrointestinal disease in the last 15 years and is becoming an essential part of the colic workup, even in the field. A 3 to 5 mHz curvilinear probe is ideal for evaluation of the equine abdomen; however information can be gained even when a higher frequency probe (such as a linear probe) is used. Imaging can be achieved with alcohol as the coupling agent, and clipping the hair is usually unnecessary. When attempting to determine the presence of a surgical lesion, focused abdominal ultrasound evaluating specific areas can be performed. A protocol for fast localized abdominal sonography of horses has been developed, which is easy to learn, quick to perform, and highly sensitive and specific for a small intestinal obstruction.[13] In this protocol, 7 sites are evaluated; however, the authors use a slightly modified protocol as described in **Table 3**.

An in-depth review on ultrasonography of the equine acute abdomen is found in the preceding article.

Abdominocentesis

The composition of the peritoneal fluid changes rapidly in response to pathophysiologic changes in the abdominal viscera. Therefore, obtaining a sample of the peritoneal fluid provides an easy and sensitive method to evaluate pathology in the

Table 3
Sites for performing a rapid focused abdominal ultrasound evaluation of horses with colic

Location	Description of Site	Normal Structures and Possible Abnormalities Identified
Ventral abdomen	Caudal to the xiphoid and at the most dependent part of the abdomen	Abdominal fluid Volume is usually minimal and any increase is considered abnormal Determination of large colon wall thickness $\geq$9 mm indicates a large colon volvulus[52]
Gastric window	Left 8–10th ICS, midway up the abdomen	Stomach Extension caudal to the 10th ICS indicates distention
Splenorenal window	Left 17th ICS in the top to middle third of the abdomen	Left kidney and spleen Gas shadowing by the colon preventing imaging of the kidney is suggestive of a nephrosplenic entrapment
Left and right inguinal areas	Lateral to sheath or mammary gland	Small intestine, colon, cecum (R). Small intestine >5 cm diameter indicates strangulation. Small intestine wall thickness >4 mm is suggestive of enteritis[53]
Duodenal window	Right side at 14–15th intercostals space on a line between the tuber coxae and elbow	Duodenum. Should contract completely Fluid distention and failure to contract is suggestive of aboral small intestinal obstruction
Right middle third	Right side, midway up the caudal abdomen	Small intestine, colon, and cecum Imaging colonic mesenteric vasculature is specific for a large colon displacement[54]
Cranial ventral thorax	Caudal to triceps muscle on left and right side	Lung Presence of free fluid indicates pleuritis

Abbreviation: ICS, Intercostal space.
   Adapted from Busoni V, De Busscher V, Lopez D, et al. Evaluation of a protocol for fast localised abdominal sonography of horses (FLASH) admitted for colic. Vet J 2011;188:78; with permission.

abdomen. The fluid sample can be obtained with either a spinal needle or a blunt ended catheter such as a bitch catheter or teat cannula.

The technique is as follows:

- Clip an approximately 3″×3″ area one hand's breadth behind the xiphoid and slightly to the right of midline just caudal to the superficial pectoral muscles. This site is usually cranial to the most dependent part of the abdomen and is more cranial than the site first described for abdominocentesis.[14]
- Aseptically prepare the area and then don sterile gloves.
- Needle technique: using an 18G 5″ spinal needle insert the needle perpendicular to midline and advance it slowly. Once the needle is situated, the stylet should be removed and the needle advanced slowly and rotated until fluid is obtained. Jerky movements of the needle indicate contact with intestinal serosa, and the needle should be withdrawn slightly and redirected.
- Cannula technique: 2 mL of local anesthetic is injected into the skin and body wall in the center of the prepared area. A #15 scalpel blade is used to create a stab incision through the skin and external rectus sheath in a transverse direction. By using this orientation a kick from the horse is less likely to accidentally result in a large cranial to caudal laceration. It is essential that the scalpel blade penetrate the external rectus sheath. Push the cannula through a sterile gauze to collect blood dripping along the outside of the cannula and prevent contamination of the sample. Push the cannula through the body wall at a perpendicular angle. After passing through the external rectus sheath, 2 "pops" should be felt, the first as the cannula penetrates the internal rectus sheath and the second as it penetrates the peritoneum. The cannula should be advanced and rotated until fluid is obtained.
- Fluid should be collected in Ethylenediaminetetraacetic acid (EDTA) and serum Vacutainer (Becton, Dickson and Company, Franklin lakes, NJ) by free catch.

Complications are rare[15] with the biggest risk being enterocentesis. Many clinicians feel that enterocentesis is more likely to occur when using a needle than a cannula. However, one study found no significant difference between the 2 techniques, with an incidence of 5.7% when a needle was used compared with 3.1% with a cannula.[16] Regardless, enterocentesis is usually inconsequential in adult horses as the hole in the bowel is small and rapidly reseals. However, enterocentesis should not be overlooked in foals because ongoing leakage from the puncture can occur, resulting in septic peritonitis. Therefore, before performing abdominocentesis in a foal it should be sedated to minimize movement during the procedure. Additionally, it is advisable to place local anesthetic at the proposed site, even when a needle is used, to minimize the likelihood of the foal reacting. Because of the risk of enterocentesis, many clinicians prefer to use a teat cannula in a foal; however, this frequently results in omentum herniating through the small stab incision in the body wall. If enterocentesis does occur in a foal, it should not be ignored and the foal should receive systemic antibiotics for 7 to 10 days to prevent septic peritonitis.

Sample analysis: changes in the peritoneal fluid occur rapidly because of the close association with the viscera. Therefore, if the results are to be meaningful and guide the decision for referral, analysis of peritoneal fluid is best performed immediately. If an abdominal fluid sample is obtained, which is abnormal based on color and/or total protein concentration, referral should be strongly considered.

- Visualization: the easiest and most useful technique for evaluation of a sample of peritoneal fluid is simply to observe the color and clarity because this alone provides extremely useful information. Normal peritoneal fluid should be yellow and transparent. A serosanguinous sample is 98% specific for a surgical lesion because red cells leach out of the devitalized bowel into the peritoneal fluid.[17] Care should be taken to ensure that this is an accurate representation of the peritoneal fluid and not merely blood contamination from the spleen or the stab incision. With blood contamination the blood will not appear to be uniformly distributed throughout the sample as it is collected.

- Total protein concentration: protein concentration can be easily read on a portable refractometer and does not require centrifugation first. The normal value is described as less than 2.5 g/dL; however, in most horses without intestinal pathology the concentration will be less than 1.5 g/dL. An elevation in protein concentration indicates an increase in the permeability of the viscera, which allows plasma protein to leak out of the circulation into the peritoneal fluid. Therefore, both medical (peritonitis) and surgical lesions can result in an elevation in protein concentration.
- Total nucleated cell count: determination of the total nucleated cell count in abdominal fluid cannot be performed immediately in the field but can be determined with simple equipment available in most practices. Nucleated cell counts in abdominal fluid are usually low at less than 5000 cells/mL. A cloudy sample is suggestive of an increased cell count. Cell counts have proved to be less reliable than color and total protein in differentiating medical and surgical colics.[17] Indeed, many surgical colic cases have nucleated cell counts in the normal range. However, rather than the total cell count, differential counts are more useful especially when performed on a cytospin smear.[18] The presence of band neutrophils or toxic changes indicates peritonitis,[18] and the sample is also inspected for the presence of bacteria or feed particles that could indicate intestinal leakage.
- Lactate: see separate section on lactate.
- Glucose: see separate section on glucose.

Lactate

High blood lactate concentrations have long been associated with a poor prognosis for colic.[9,19] Lactate can be measured in the field using small portable lactate meters, with results being obtained within 10 to 60 seconds. Several models are available (Lactate Scout, EKF Diagnostics, Accutrend, Roche, Lactate Pro 2, Arkray) and all have proved to accurately measure lactate in equine blood.[20–22] Because these lactate meters provide rapid, easy, and cheap methods to determine lactate concentration, measurement of blood and abdominal fluid lactate has become one of the most helpful techniques to determine the degree of circulatory and intestinal compromise in horses with colic.

Blood lactate concentration is usually less than 1.5 mmol/L. Physical exertion in horses with colic may result in elevations from 2 to 3 mmol based on the authors' experience. However, blood lactate concentrations greater than 3 mmol/L are usually associated with the presence of ischemic intestine. Blood lactate concentration may be particularly helpful in determining the potential prognosis in horses with large colon volvulus. Blood lactate at hospital admission in horses with large colon volvulus was compared to survival. If blood lactate was less than 6 mmol/L, 90% of horses survived compared with only 30% survival if lactate concentration was greater than 7 mmol/L.[23] Care should be taken when interpreting blood lactate concentration in ponies because lactate values are significantly higher, even in ponies with nonsurgical lesions, than in horses.[24]

For horses with a suspected small intestinal lesion, comparison of blood and peritoneal fluid lactate concentrations can help identify the presence of ischemic-injured intestine. In normal horses, peritoneal lactate is lower than plasma lactate at approximately 0.7 mmol/L. Horses with nonstrangulating obstructions have peritoneal fluid lactate values of approximately 2 mmol/L.[25] Ischemic segments of intestine rapidly leak small molecules such as lactate into the peritoneal fluid. This results in a rapid elevation in peritoneal fluid lactate, whereas blood lactate does not rise so rapidly while the horse is systemically stable. Therefore, an elevated peritoneal fluid lactate compared with blood lactate is a sensitive indicator for the presence of ischemic intestine[25] and the need for referral for emergency surgery. If the need for referral remains in doubt, a second abdominal fluid sample can be obtained 1 to 6 hours after the first and the results of the 2 samples compared. An elevation in peritoneal lactate compared with the first sample is highly suggestive of the progression of ischemia and the need for referral for surgery.[26]

A complete discussion on the utility of lactate in critically ill adults and neonates is found in the next article.

Glucose

Hyperglycemia is common in horses with colic and is associated with a poor prognosis. Conversely, hypoglycemia is rarely identified in adult horses with colic. Blood glucose concentration becomes dysregulated due to the action of endotoxin, which is absorbed across compromised intestinal mucosa and causes insulin resistance and hence an elevation in blood glucose concentration.[27] Blood glucose concentration is measured rapidly and easily in the field using a handheld glucometer. However, there is poor correlation in glucose concentration when testing whole blood with a human glucometer and plasma chemistry analyzer results for horses.[28] A veterinary glucometer (AlphaTRAK 2, Abbott Animal Health), which accounts for the higher percentage of glucose in the plasma of veterinary species, may be more accurate.[29] Care should be taken in interpreting glucose concentrations after an alpha-2 agonist has been administered because these sedatives cause hyperglycemia.[30]

Approximately 50% of horses with colic admitted to referral hospitals are hyperglycemic (>135 mg/dL).[31,32] Hyperglycemia in the horse with colic may indicate the presence of devitalized intestine and the need for referral. Extreme hyperglycemia (>180 mg/dL) in adult horses with colic has been associated with[31,32]

- Surgical colic
- Strangulating small intestinal lesions that require resection
- Decrease in hospital survival
- Decreased survival in the first 100 days after hospitalization

Glucose concentration can also be measured in peritoneal fluid with a glucometer. Blood and peritoneal fluid glucose concentrations are usually tightly correlated with peritoneal glucose concentrations being slightly higher than those in blood.[33] If bacteria are present in peritoneal fluid they use glucose and result in a lower glucose concentration in peritoneal fluid compared with blood. Therefore, peritoneal fluid glucose concentrations are low in horses with septic peritonitis, and this is a useful test to perform if the abdominal fluid is cloudy and hence there is a suspicion of peritonitis. Peritoneal fluid glucose concentrations less than 30 mg/dL are 100% specific for septic peritonitis.[34] Using the absolute value for peritoneal fluid glucose as the determining factor is not very sensitive, however, because some horses with septic peritonitis may have profound hyperglycemia and hence peritoneal glucose concentrations greater than 30 mg/dL. In such situations the specificity of this test is increased further if the serum and peritoneal glucose concentrations are compared. If peritoneal fluid glucose concentration is greater than 50 mg/dL less than blood glucose concentration, a diagnosis of septic peritonitis can be made, even if the absolute concentration is greater than 30 mg/dL.

Overall the measurement of peritoneal fluid glucose concentration can be used as follows:

- Perform this test if peritoneal fluid is cloudy
- Concentration less than 30 mg/dL indicates septic peritonitis
- Concentration greater than 30 mg/dL should be compared with blood glucose concentration:
  - Blood glucose concentration greater than 50 mg/dL higher than peritoneal glucose concentration indicates septic peritonitis
  - Blood glucose concentration less than 50 mg/dL higher than peritoneal glucose concentration suggests nonseptic peritonitis
- Results are used to guide initial therapy; however, a full fluid cytology should be performed to confirm the diagnosis

SUMMARY

A thorough evaluation of the horse with colic is critical during the first visit to identify the small number of cases that would benefit from referral. Physical examination, including rectal examination and passage of a nasogastric tube to determine if there is gastric distention, are the foundation of this evaluation. More advanced diagnostic tests, including transabdominal ultrasound, abdominocentesis, and point-of-care measurement of lactate and glucose in blood and peritoneal fluid, can aid in determining if referral should be offered to the client. If doubt still exists, referral will allow further diagnostics to be performed along with around the clock monitoring to determine if advanced medical or surgical intervention is required.

REFERENCES

1. Traub-Dargatz JL, Kopral CA, Seitzinger AH, et al. Estimate of the national incidence of and operation-level risk factors for colic among horses in the United States, spring 1998 to spring 1999. J Am Vet Med Assoc 2001;219:67–71.
2. Proudman CJ. A two year, prospective survey of equine colic in general practice. Equine Vet J 1992;24:90–3.
3. Southwood LL, Gassert T, Lindborg S. Colic in geriatric compared to mature nongeriatric horses. Part 2: treatment, diagnosis and short-term survival. Equine Vet J 2010;42:628–35.
4. Pratt SM, Hassel DM. Clinical characteristics of horses with gastrointestinal ruptures revealed during initial diagnostic evaluation: 149 cases (1990-2002). 49th Annual Convention of the American Association of Equine Practitioners. New Orleans (LA): 21–25 November, 2003. p. 366–70.
5. Ducharme NG, Lowe JE. Decision for surgery. Vet Clin North Am Equine Pract 1988;4:51–61.
6. White NA, Elward A, Moga KS, et al. Use of web-based data collection to evaluate analgesic administration and the decision for surgery in horses with colic. Equine Vet J 2005;37:347–50.
7. Husted L, Andersen MS, Borggaard OK, et al. Risk factors for faecal sand excretion in Icelandic horses. Equine Vet J 2005;37:351–5.

8. Furr MO, Lessard P, White NA 2nd. Development of a colic severity score for predicting the outcome of equine colic. Vet Surg 1995;24:97–101.

9. Orsini JA, Elser AH, Galligan DT, et al. Prognostic index for acute abdominal crisis (colic) in horses. Am J Vet Res 1988;49:1969–71.

10. Reeves MJ, Curtis CR, Salman MD, et al. Prognosis in equine colic patients using multivariable analysis. Can J Vet Res 1989;53:87–94.

11. Morton AJ, Varney CR, Ekiri AB, et al. Cardiovascular effects of N-butylscopolammonium bromide and xylazine in horses. Equine Vet J Suppl 2011;43:117–22.

12. Underwood C, Southwood LL, McKeown LP, et al. Complications and survival associated with surgical compared with medical management of horses with duodenitis-proximal jejunitis. Equine Vet J 2008;40:373–8.

13. Busoni V, De Busscher V, Lopez D, et al. Evaluation of a protocol for fast localised abdominal sonography of horses (FLASH) admitted for colic. Vet J 2011; 188:77–82.

14. Bach LG, Ricketts SW. Paracentesis as an aid to the diagnosis of abdominal disease in the horse. Equine Vet J 1974;6:116–21.

15. Tulleners EP. Complications of abdominocentesis in the horse. J Am Vet Med Assoc 1983;182:232–4.

16. Siex MT, Wilson JH. Morbidity associated with abdominocentesis - A prospective study. Equine Vet J Suppl 1992;13:23–5.

17. Matthews S, Dart AJ, Reid SW, et al. Predictive values, sensitivity and specificity of abdominal fluid variables in determining the need for surgery in horses with an acute abdominal crisis. Aust Vet J 2002;80:132–6.

18. Garma-Avina A. Cytology of 100 samples of abdominal fluid from 100 horses with abdominal disease. Equine Vet J 1998;30:435–44.

19. Moore JN, Owen RR, Lumsden JH. Clinical evaluation of blood lactate levels in equine colic. Equine Vet J 1976;8:49–54.

20. Sloet van Oldruitenborgh-Oosterbaan MM, van den Broek ET, Spierenburg AJ. Evaluation of the usefulness of the portable device Lactate Pro for measurement of lactate concentrations in equine whole blood. J Vet Diagn Invest 2008;20: 83–5.

21. Tennent-Brown BS, Wilkins PA, Lindborg S, et al. Assessment of a point-of-care lactate monitor in emergency admissions of adult horses to a referral hospital. J Vet Intern Med 2007;21:1090–8.

22. Castagnetti C, Pirrone A, Mariella J, et al. Venous blood lactate evaluation in equine neonatal intensive care. Theriogenology 2010;73:343–57.

23. Johnston K, Holcombe SJ, Hauptman JG. Plasma lactate as a predictor of colonic viability and survival after 360 degrees volvulus of the ascending colon in horses. Vet Surg 2007;36:563–7.

24. Dunkel B, Kapff JE, Naylor RJ, et al. Blood lactate concentrations in ponies and miniature horses with gastrointestinal disease. Equine Vet J 2013;45:666–70.

25. Latson KM, Nieto JE, Beldomenico PM, et al. Evaluation of peritoneal fluid lactate as a marker of intestinal ischaemia in equine colic. Equine Vet J 2005;37:342–6.

26. Peloso JG, Cohen ND. Use of serial measurements of peritoneal fluid lactate concentration to identify strangulating intestinal lesions in referred horses with signs of colic. J Am Vet Med Assoc 2012;240:1208–17.

27. Toth F, Frank N, Chameroy KA, et al. Effects of endotoxaemia and carbohydrate overload on glucose and insulin dynamics and the development of laminitis in horses. Equine Vet J 2009;41:852–8.

28. Hollis AR, Dallap Schaer BL, Boston RC, et al. Comparison of the Accu-Chek Aviva point-of-care glucometer with blood gas and laboratory methods of analysis

of glucose measurement in equine emergency patients. J Vet Intern Med 2008;22: 1189–95.

29. Hackett ES, McCue PM. Evaluation of a veterinary glucometer for use in horses. J Vet Intern Med 2010;24:617–21.

30. Thurmon JC, Steffey EP, Zinkl JG, et al. Xylazine causes transient dose-related hyperglycemia and increased urine volumes in mares. Am J Vet Res 1984;45: 224–7.

31. Hassel DM, Hill AE, Rorabeck RA. Association between hyperglycemia and survival in 228 horses with acute gastrointestinal disease. J Vet Intern Med 2009;23: 1261–5.

32. Hollis AR, Boston RC, Corley KT. Blood glucose in horses with acute abdominal disease. J Vet Intern Med 2007;21:1099–103.

33. Brownlow MA, Hutchins DR, Johnston KG. Reference values for equine peritoneal fluid. Equine Vet J 1981;13:127–30.

34. Van Hoogmoed L, Rodger LD, Spier SJ, et al. Evaluation of peritoneal fluid pH, glucose concentration, and lactate dehydrogenase activity for detection of septic peritonitis in horses. J Am Vet Med Assoc 1999;214:1032–6.

35. Frederico LM, Jones SL, Blikslager AT. Predisposing factors for small colon impaction in horses and outcome of medical and surgical treatment: 44 cases (1999-2004). J Am Vet Med Assoc 2006;229:1612–6.

36. Hillyer MH, Taylor FG, Proudman CJ, et al. Case control study to identify risk factors for simple colonic obstruction and distension colic in horses. Equine Vet J 2002;34:455–63.

37. Hudson JM, Cohen ND, Gibbs PG, et al. Feeding practices associated with colic in horses. J Am Vet Med Assoc 2001;219:1419–25.

38. Cohen ND, Toby E, Roussel AJ, et al. Are feeding practices associated with duodenitis-proximal jejunitis? Equine Vet J 2006;38:526–31.

39. Hassel DM, Langer DL, Snyder JR, et al. Evaluation of enterolithiasis in equids: 900 cases (1973-1996). J Am Vet Med Assoc 1999;214:233–7.

40. Southwood LL, Baxter GM, Bennett DG, et al. Ascarid impaction in young horses. Compendium on Continuing Education for the Practicing Veterinarian 1998;20:100–6.

41. McConnico RS, Morgan TW, Williams CC, et al. Pathophysiologic effects of phenylbutazone on the right dorsal colon in horses. Am J Vet Res 2008;69:1496–505.

42. McCarthy HE, Proudman CJ, French NP. Epidemiology of equine grass sickness: a literature review. Vet Rec 2001;149:293–300.

43. Boles CL, Kohn CW. Fibrous foreign body impaction colic in young horses. J Am Vet Med Assoc 1977;171:193–5.

44. Cribb NC, Cote NM, Boure LP, et al. Acute small intestinal obstruction associated with Parascaris equorum infection in young horses: 25 cases (1985-2004). N Z Vet J 2006;54:338–43.

45. Martin BB Jr, Freeman DE, Ross MW, et al. Cecocolic and cecocecal intussusception in horses: 30 cases (1976-1996). J Am Vet Med Assoc 1999;214:80–4.

46. Haupt JL, McAndrews AG, Chaney KP, et al. Surgical treatment of colic in the miniature horse: a retrospective study of 57 cases (1993-2006). Equine Vet J 2008;40:364–7.

47. Cohen ND, Vontur CA, Rakestraw PC. Risk factors for enterolithiasis among horses in Texas. J Am Vet Med Assoc 2000;216:1787–94.

48. Munoz E, Arguelles D, Areste L, et al. Retrospective analysis of exploratory laparotomies in 192 Andalusian horses and 276 horses of other breeds. Vet Rec 2008;162:303–6.

49. Schneider RK, Milne DW, Kohn CW. Acquired inguinal hernia in the horse: a review of 27 cases. J Am Vet Med Assoc 1982;180:317–20.
50. Carmalt JL, Shoemaker RW, Wilson DG. Evaluation of common vaginal tunic ligation during field castration in draught colts. Equine Vet J 2008;40:597–8.
51. Ueno T, Nambo Y, Tajima Y, et al. Pathology of lethal peripartum broad ligament haematoma in 31 Thoroughbred mares. Equine Vet J 2010;42:529–33.
52. Pease AP, Scrivani PV, Erb HN, et al. Accuracy of increased large-intestine wall thickness during ultrasonography for diagnosing large-colon torsion in 42 horses. Vet Radiol Ultrasound 2004;45:220–4.
53. Freeman SL. Ultrasonography of the equine abdomen: findings in the colic patient. Practice 2002;24:262–73.
54. Ness SL, Bain FT, Zantingh AJ, et al. Ultrasonographic visualization of colonic mesenteric vasculature as an indicator of large colon right dorsal displacement or 180 degrees volvulus (or both) in horses. Can Vet J 2012;53:378–82.

Blood Lactate Measurement and Interpretation in Critically Ill Equine Adults and Neonates

Brett Tennent-Brown, BVSc, MS

KEYWORDS

- Equine • Lactate • Serial measurement • Lactate clearance

KEY POINTS

- Increases in blood lactate concentration in horses are usually the result of decreased tissue perfusion and oxygen delivery. However, other mechanisms for hyperlactatemia exist and might be important in some critically ill horses.
- Lactate concentrations measured at hospital admission are a useful prognostic guide but there are limitations to its interpretation. Serial lactate measurement or measurement of lactate clearance might improve prognostic usefulness.
- Serial lactate measurement might be a useful guide for therapeutic interventions, particularly early (resuscitative) fluid therapy.

INTRODUCTION

Lactate exists as L-isomers and D-isomers; L-lactate is the stereoisomer produced by mammalian cells and the focus of this review. D-Lactate is primarily a product of bacterial carbohydrate metabolism and is not discussed further, although it is important in some disease conditions, especially in ruminants.[1] L-Lactate has historically been considered a marker of tissue hypoxia and a dead-end product of carbohydrate metabolism. These concepts have required extensive reevaluation over the past 25 years. Hyperlactatemia can occur in the presence of apparently adequate tissue perfusion and oxygen delivery.[2,3] Lactate can act as an alternative energy source for the brain during cerebral ischemia and the heart during hemorrhagic shock.[4,5] Rather than a dead-end product, lactate is an important carbohydrate intermediate, which is

Funding Sources: None.
Conflict of Interest: None.
Faculty of Veterinary Science, Equine Centre, The University of Melbourne, 250 Princess Highway, Werribee, Victoria 3030, Australia
E-mail address: brett.tennent@unimelb.edu.au

shuttled between tissues.[6] Lactate might even have a role in cell signaling![7] Blood (or plasma) lactate concentration at hospital admission has proved to be a useful indicator of disease severity, but measurements taken at a single time point typically fail to completely discriminate survivors from nonsurvivors. Measures that reflect both the severity and duration of hyperlactatemia in critically ill patients might provide better prognostic information. However, the true value of serial blood lactate measurements may lie in its role as a therapeutic target.

MEASURING LACTATE CONCENTRATIONS

In the blood, lactate is present both in plasma and within erythrocytes[8,9]; plasma lactate concentrations are most commonly measured, but whole blood lactate concentrations might be more appropriate in some situations. Measurement of whole blood lactate concentration requires erythrolysis and is a weighted average of plasma and intraerythrocyte lactate concentrations. Most clinical lactate measuring devices report plasma concentrations, although whole blood samples are used in some, making them, at least theoretically, more convenient. The methodologies routinely used to measure lactate are isomer specific and detect only L-lactate. In most healthy mammals, the D-isomer exists only in nanomolar concentrations, and special assays are required to determine D-lactate concentrations.[10]

Inexpensive, handheld point of care (POC) meters have become popular in human critical care medicine, because they can decrease analytical time and cost. Many of these meters are also widely used in equine medicine, although only a few have been validated for use in the horse.[11–16] The fact that whole blood rather than plasma samples are used in many of these devices has implications for both the accuracy and interpretation of lactate measurements. One POC meter designed to measure plasma lactate concentrations in humans using whole blood samples was assessed in adult horses admitted for emergency assessment and treatment.[11] When using plasma samples, lactate concentrations reported by the POC meter correlated well with values obtained using a standard laboratory-based method. However, the meter could be relatively inaccurate when whole blood samples were used; at lower lactate concentrations (<5 mmol/L), the meter commonly overestimates lactate concentrations by 1 or 2 mmol/L.[11] Although this discrepancy might seem inconsequential, it can become clinically relevant when assessing animals with near normal lactate concentrations.

The causes of this inaccuracy are unknown, but similar issues have been reported for handheld glucometers evaluated in horses[17] and other species.[18] Packed cell volume seems to be a factor in some studies, and the algorithms used to calculate plasma lactate concentration in human whole blood samples might not be appropriate for equine samples.[11] Equine erythrocytes might also physically interfere with meter function, perhaps because of their rapid sedimentation.

Patient and sample handling can also have clinically important effects on the measurement of blood lactate concentrations. Arterial versus venous sampling has some effect on the measured lactate concentration, but the differences are typically clinically irrelevant[19]; venous samples are obviously more convenient to collect and give a better overview of the metabolic status of a patient. Blood lactate concentrations can be increased in struggling animals (or animals that are difficult to capture), and prolonged occlusion of the vessel might cause a slight increase in the lactate concentration.[20] Inadequate clearance of lactate-containing fluids (eg, lactated Ringer's solution) from intravenous catheters may falsely increase the measured lactate concentration.[20] Conversely, fluids that do not contain lactate might falsely decrease lactate concentrations if not completely flushed from the intravenous catheter during sample collection.[20] Erythrocytes are obligate lactate producers and continue to produce lactate ex vivo if samples are not stored appropriately. Lactate concentration in whole blood samples kept at room temperature can change considerably and unpredictably even over a short period.[21] Shuttling of lactate between plasma and erythrocytes might contribute to this situation in samples that are not analyzed immediately. Ideally, samples should be analyzed within 5 to 10 minutes of collection; if a delay of more than 10 minutes before analysis is expected, samples should be collected into tubes containing sodium fluoride–potassium oxalate and chilled (0°C–4°C [32°F–39.2°F]).[21] Sodium fluoride–potassium oxalate combinations inhibit several glycolytic enzymes, preventing lactate production; however, sodium fluoride also causes erythrolysis and affects the measurement of glucose concentrations.[21]

LACTATE METABOLISM IN THE HEALTHY ANIMAL

Adenosine 5'-triphosphate (ATP) is the primary source of energy of the cell and is generated from the metabolism of glucose in 2 sequential pathways. The first of these pathways is glycolysis; glycolysis is then followed by the citric acid (Krebs or tricarboxylic acid) cycle during aerobic conditions. Intermediates produced by the citric acid cycle enter the electron transport chain for oxidative phosphorylation, where most ATP is generated. Glycolysis is a 10-step, cytosolic process, which converts a single molecule of glucose into 2 molecules of pyruvate. This sequence of reactions does not require oxygen (ie, it is anaerobic) but is inefficient, generating only 2 molecules of ATP for every molecule of glucose. In comparison, reactions within the mitochondria (ie, the citric acid cycle and oxidative phosphorylation) generate 34 molecules of ATP for every molecule of glucose metabolized. In the presence of oxygen, pyruvate is converted to acetyl coenzyme A (acetyl co-A) by the enzyme pyruvate dehydrogenase (PDH) for metabolism within the citric acid cycle. However, in the absence of oxygen, pyruvate is unable to enter the mitochondria, and the cell must rely entirely on glycolysis to generate ATP.

Under anaerobic conditions, pyruvate is preferentially transformed into lactate. The conversion of pyruvate to lactate regenerates the nicotinamide adenine dinucleotide that is needed for continued glycolysis and ATP production. Because it is less efficient, the rate of glycolysis must increase dramatically during anaerobiosis to produce enough ATP to maintain cellular function. The conversion of pyruvate to lactate consumes rather than produces H^+ ions. It is the increased rate of glycolysis and the cytosolic (ie, nonmitochondrial) hydrolysis of ATP to adenosine diphosphate that is responsible for the increase in H^+ ion concentration and acidosis that typically accompanies anaerobic metabolism.[22]

Although some of the cells of the body periodically operate under anaerobic conditions, others (eg, erythrocytes) lack mitochondria and the enzymes required to metabolize pyruvate and are, consequently, obligate lactate producers.[23] The average human produces lactate at a rate of approximately 0.8 mmol/kg/h[24] and, based on the clearance of exogenously administered lactate, lactate production by healthy horses is 0.53 ± 0.24 mmol/kg/h.[25] The organs producing most lactate under normal conditions are the skin, erythrocytes, and skeletal muscles.[23] Lactate is primarily metabolized by the liver, which converts approximately 50% to 70% of plasma lactate to pyruvate; the liver is also able to increase its rate of lactate metabolism if required. Most pyruvate derived from hepatic lactate metabolism is directed to the citric acid cycle for oxidation or the Cori cycle for gluconeogenesis. The renal cortex and skeletal muscle account for the remainder of plasma lactate metabolism, and renal consumption might become more important during sepsis.[26] Lactate is not excreted in the urine until plasma concentrations exceed 6 to 10 mmol/L.

LACTATE METABOLISM IN DISEASE

Hyperlactatemia can be categorized as either type A or type B.[27] Type A hyperlactatemia occurs with a relative or absolute deficit in tissue oxygenation, whereas type B occurs when tissue oxygenation is maintained (**Table 1**).[27] Type B hyperlactatemia has been further divided into 3 subtypes: type B_1 is associated with an underlying disease process; B_2 with drugs or toxins; and B_3 is hyperlactatemia caused by congenital metabolic defects.[28] Clinical experience suggests that the hyperlactatemia caused by type B causes are usually mild to moderate (2–3 mmol/L). Moderate to severe hyperlactatemia (>6 mmol/L) is typically caused by global hypoperfusion and type A causes. Type A and B hyperlactatemia occur concurrently in some patients and this might be common during sepsis.

Decreased bulk oxygen delivery with subsequent tissue hypoxia and anaerobiosis is probably the most common cause of increased blood lactate concentrations in critically ill horses; that is, most horses have a type A hyperlactatemia.[29] Some of the postulated mechanisms for type B hyperlactatemia are discussed in the following sections. The underlying lesion in many of these cases is an intense inflammatory reaction.

Increased Na+/K+–Adenosine Triphosphatase Activity in Response to Inflammatory Mediators

Increased plasma catecholamine concentrations, particularly epinephrine, during septic (and hemorrhagic) shock indirectly increase activity of the Na^+/K^+–adenosine triphosphatase (ATPase) pumps located on the cell membrane.[30] As a consequence of the increased pump activity, the rate of glycolysis must increase to meet energy (ATP) requirements. Na^+/K^+-ATPase pumps have a dedicated set of glycolytic enzymes, which are not shared with those of the cellular energy metabolism apparatus. Pyruvate produced by pump-associated glycolytic enzymes is not fed into the citric acid cycle but is preferentially converted to lactate and subsequently exported from the cell.[30] Studies have shown that muscle glycogen was the ultimate

---

Table 1
Selected causes of type A and B hyperlactatemia

Type A	Type B
Decreased Oxygen Delivery	B_1: Hyperlactatemia Associated with Underlying Disease
Hypotension	Sepsis/systemic inflammatory response syndrome
Hypovolemia	Liver disease
Blood loss	Parenteral nutrition (hyperglycemia?)
Cardiogenic shock	Diabetes mellitus
Septic shock	Malignancy
Severe anemia	Thiamine deficiency
Severe hypoxemia	B_2: Hyperlactatemia Associated with Drugs or Toxins
Carbon monoxide poisoning	Propylene glycol
Increased Oxygen Demand	Bicarbonate
Exercise	Catecholamines
Seizures	B_3: Hyperlactatemia Associated with Mitochondrial
Shivering	Dysfunction

Data from Refs.[19,20,27,28]

source of lactate, suggesting that skeletal muscle is a major source of lactate during sepsis.

Inhibition of PDH

PDH is the enzyme responsible for conversion of pyruvate to acetyl co-A within the mitochondria and a key regulator of glucose metabolism. PDH activity is increased by the action of PDH phosphatase and decreased by PDH kinase.[31] A decrease in PDH activity favors conversion of pyruvate to lactate rather than to acetyl co-A. Skeletal muscle PDH activity was reduced in experimental sepsis induced by placing a fecal-agar pellet inoculated with *Escherichia coli* and *Bacteroides fragilis* within the peritoneal cavity of rats.[32] Sterile inflammation did not alter PDH activity, suggesting that bacterial products were required for the inhibitory effect. Decreased PDH activity in this model is believed to be mediated via increased PDH kinase activity.[31] Dichloroacetate (DCA) is a halogenated hydrocarbon that indirectly stimulates PDH complex activity, accelerating the oxidation of lactate via pyruvate. DCA reduces hyperlactatemia in a range of disease conditions, including sepsis, lending support to the suggestion that PDH inhibition contributes to hyperlactatemia in sepsis.[33,34] Although DCA can reduce lactate concentrations (and the accompanying acidosis), outcome is often not improved with administration, underlining the fact that hyperlactatemia is likely more a marker of disease pathogenesis rather than a contributor to morbidity and mortality.[33]

Lactate Production by Leukocytes

Approximately 80% of glucose metabolized by inflammatory leukocytes is converted to lactate. It has been suggested[35] that lactate production by inflammatory cells sequestered within tissue beds might, at least in part, account for the hyperlactatemia encountered in sepsis. In a rat cecal ligation and puncture model, lactate production by peritoneal leukocytes was increased when compared with leukocytes isolated from control (sham operated) rats. In addition, ex vivo lactate production by leukocytes isolated from human intensive care patients after lipopolysaccharide stimulation was higher when compared with leukocytes isolated from healthy people.[35] On a wet weight basis, leukocytes can produce more lactate than tissues traditionally considered to be lactate producers (ie, skeletal muscle, intestine).

Inflammatory cell metabolism (rather than bacterial metabolism) is likely the cause of the increased lactate (and decreased glucose) concentrations seen in inflammatory exudates in peritonitis, pleuritis, and septic arthritis. In contrast, the increase in lactate concentration in the peritoneal fluid from animals with ischemic gastrointestinal lesions likely reflects anaerobic metabolism by the strangulated bowel.[36,37]

Decreased Hepatic Clearance

Because the liver is the primary organ responsible for lactate metabolism, it has been suggested[38] that hepatocellular injury or decreased hepatic perfusion might contribute to hyperlactatemia during sepsis. In hemodynamically stable septic patients with hyperlactatemia (≥2 mmol/L), blood lactate concentration returned more slowly to baseline after infusion of exogenous lactate when compared with stable, septic patients with normal blood lactate concentrations (≤1.5 mmol/L), suggesting impaired hepatic clearance.[39] However, hepatic extraction of lactate was increased rather than decreased in rats during lipopolysaccharide infusion,[40] and lactate clearance in human patients with septic or cardiogenic shock was similar to that measured in healthy volunteers.[41] In patients with multiple-system organ failure but without obvious hepatic involvement, the hepatosplanchnic region (ie, liver and gastrointestinal tract) cleared, rather than produced, lactate.[42] The role of the liver in hyperlactatemia during sepsis is, therefore, unclear and likely varies between patients. However, it seems reasonable to assume that impaired hepatic clearance could contribute to hyperlactatemia in patients with severe liver failure.

Other Potential Causes of Hyperlactatemia

Other causes of hyperlactatemia during aerobic conditions include impaired mitochondrial function,[43] hypermetabolism and increased tissue glycolysis,[44] propylene glycol toxicity,[45] and administration of exogenous catecholamines (epinephrine and norepinephrine).[27,46,47] Administration of sodium bicarbonate is associated with increases in blood lactate concentration under some circumstances.[48,49] Increases in blood lactate concentration are occasionally observed after aggressive fluid resuscitation of extremely hypovolemic patients and are presumably the result of lactate washout as tissue perfusion is reestablished. Hyperlactatemia has also been associated with some forms of hematologic malignancies in human and veterinary medicine, because some neoplastic cells have high rates of glycolysis and consequently produce lactate.[50,51]

Source of Lactate During Disease

Studies investigating the role of increased Na^+/K^+-ATPase activity[30,52,53] and impaired PDH activity[32,54] in hyperlactatemia have indicated that skeletal muscle is the most important source of lactate during severe illness. It has also been suggested that the lungs and splanchnic tissues might become significant lactate producers in some critically ill patients.[38,55,56] Production of lactate by pulmonary tissues does increase in some patients with severe acute lung injury, and increased lactate production by the splanchnic tissues has described.[41,56,57] The mechanism of increased tissue lactate production has not been elucidated but might be caused by increased tissue glycolysis, microvascular injury (and subsequent focal tissue hypoxia), or leukocyte sequestration. However, the arteriovenous difference in lactate concentrations is small in most studies, and the contribution of splanchnic or pulmonary lactate production to global hyperlactatemia is probably negligible.[57] Microvascular injury and local hypoperfusion might result in increased regional lactate production but the effect on global lactate concentrations is difficult to predict. Experimental ischemia of a 40-cm section of colon for 1 hour caused a marked (but transient) increase in the lactate concentration measured in the draining colonic vein.[58] However, there was little or no effect on lactate concentrations measured in jugular venous samples.[58] This finding suggests that increases in peripheral lactate concentration in horses with ischemic gastrointestinal lesions are a result of global hypoperfusion rather than increased lactate production by the section of ischemic bowel.[36]

INTERPRETATION OF BLOOD LACTATE CONCENTRATIONS IN CRITICALLY ILL HORSES

Numerous studies in human and veterinary medicine have documented a significant association between outcome and blood lactate concentration. Mortality (or morbidity) typically increases with increasing blood lactate concentration when measured at hospital admission or transfer to the intensive care unit. However, some studies have been unable to find a significant association between lactate concentration and outcome. In addition, there is invariably considerable overlap in admission lactate concentrations between (for example) survivors and nonsurvivors, which limits its value in determining prognosis. The reasons that lactate concentrations measured at a single time point might perform poorly as a prognostic indicator are many and varied. The underlying disease process driving the hyperlactatemia undoubtedly has a profound effect on the significance of a patient's blood lactate concentration.[59] Lactate metabolism is a dynamic process, so the timing of sample collection in relationship to disease onset, the severity of disease, and whether any treatments have been administered before sample collection also almost certainly affects interpretation.

Serial lactate measurement might better reflect the magnitude and duration of hyperlactatemia and allow more accurate prognostication. In human critical care medicine, serial lactate measurement seems to more accurately predict outcome than a single measurement. Persistent hyperlactatemia in the face of appropriate treatment is associated with lower survival rates and a higher incidence of multiple organ failure in human patients.[60–62] Several studies in horses have shown that the risk of nonsurvival increases considerably for the same unit increase in blood lactate concentration over the course of hospitalization; that is, the clinical significance of hyperlactatemia becomes greater later in hospitalization when compared with admission.[29,63]

Measures of lactate clearance might reflect either the underlying disease process or the patient's ability to compensate for increased lactate production. Lactate clearance might aid in prognostication but, perhaps more importantly, could provide insight into disease pathogenesis. Crude indices of lactate clearance have been investigated in equine medicine.[29,63,64] Values for exogenous lactate clearance have now been determined in normal adult horses, which allows more thorough evaluation of the mechanism or mechanisms for hyperlactatemia in critically ill horses.[25]

Whether serial lactate measurements or measures of lactate clearance improve the clinician's ability to accurately estimate prognosis remains to be determined. However, the true worth of lactate might be as a resuscitation target; with the advent of inexpensive, accurate lactate meters many clinicians are finding value in using blood lactate concentration to guide fluid therapy, particularly in the acute phase. However, there is little or no evidence that the use of blood lactate concentrations to guide therapy in critically ill horses improves outcome.

Lactate Measurement and Interpretation in Adult Horses

The measurement of blood lactate concentrations in adult horses has received the most attention in evaluating horses with a primary complaint of colic.[36,65–69] Studies dating back to the mid-1970s have confirmed a statistically significant association between increasing blood lactate concentrations at hospital admission and decreased survival to discharge.[36,65,67,69] A study that measured blood lactate concentrations in 250 horses presenting to a university referral hospital for emergency treatment (including 152 horses with colic) found that the odds ratio (OR) for nonsurvival increased by 29% for every 1 mmol/L increase in admission blood (plasma) lactate concentration.[29] Earlier studies suggested that the probability of survival decreased substantially once blood lactate concentration exceeded 4 to 6 mmol/L.[36,69] With improvements in equine medicine and surgery over the last 30 years, this range is perhaps slightly pessimistic. Clinical experience suggests that prognosis worsens considerably once blood lactate concentration exceeds 6 to 8 mmol/L, and horses with lactate concentrations greater than 8 to 10 mmol/L probably have a guarded prognosis. These divisions are, of course, arbitrary; lactate concentrations must be considered in light of the underlying disease and other clinical and clinical pathologic findings. It has been reported that ponies (and miniature horse breeds) with gastrointestinal disease have higher blood lactate concentrations at admission when compared with large breed horses with disease of similar severity.[70] The reasons for this difference are not known, but clinicians should perhaps temper their predictions when evaluating admission lactate concentrations in ponies. In addition, a recent retrospective study evaluating horses with colitis found no association between admission lactate concentration and outcome.[64] There is probably not a lactate concentration (within reason) beyond which survival is hopeless.

The usefulness of serial or sequential measurement of blood lactate concentrations has been investigated in a few equine studies.[29,63,64,71,72] As in human patients, horses in which lactate concentration remains increased or decreases slowly in the face of appropriate therapy have poorer outcomes. In adult horses diagnosed with a large colon volvulus, mean ($\pm$ standard deviation [SD]) lactate concentration returned to normal 24 hours postoperatively in survivors (0.96 $\pm$ 0.06 mmol/L) but remained increased in nonsurvivors (3.24 $\pm$ 2.08 mmol/L).[73] In 250 horses evaluated prospectively with a range of emergent conditions, blood lactate concentrations were significantly higher in nonsurvivors at all time points, although the difference beyond 12 hours of hospital admission was subtle.[29] Similar results were reported in a recent study evaluating horses requiring emergency abdominal surgery.[72] The OR for nonsurvival increased considerably for every unit increase in lactate concentration over the course of hospitalization in 1 study.[29] At admission, the OR for nonsurvival was 1.29 (95% confidence interval 1.17–1.43) for every 1 mmol/L increase in lactate concentration; by 72 hours after admission the OR for nonsurvival had increased to 49.90 (95% confidence interval 6.47–384.82).[29] Using a crude index of lactate clearance, lactate concentrations tended to decrease more rapidly in nonsurviving horses over the first 12 to 24 hours of hospitalization, suggesting that lactate clearance mechanisms were intact, at least initially, in those horses.[29] However, between 24 and 72 hours after admission, lactate concentrations increased subtly but significantly in nonsurvivors compared with survivors.[29] Further studies are required to determine whether this increase in lactate concentration is a result of increased production or decreased metabolism.[25] Although admission lactate concentration was not associated with outcome in a study examining horses with colitis, a decrease in lactate concentration of 30% or higher by 4 to 8 hours after admission or a decrease of 50% or higher by 24 hours after admission was associated with survival.[64]

Although optimal sampling times, duration of sampling, and targets (or cut points) remain to be defined, serial lactate measurements might enable better discrimination between survivors and nonsurvivors. However, the true benefit of serial lactate measurement likely lies in monitoring the response to therapy, particularly during early fluid resuscitation. The availability of inexpensive, accurate meters that provide real-time results allows clinicians to frequently monitor lactate concentrations and tailor therapy accordingly. The optimal rate of decrease in lactate concentration is not known, but most horses should have a lactate concentration less than 1.5 mmol/L within 6 to 12 hours of initiating therapy.[29,64,72] However, some surviving horses might not achieve this goal within 72 hours of admission. Based on results in horses with colitis, other targets might include a reduction in lactate concentration by at least 30% 4 to 8 hours after admission or at least 50% by 24 hours after admission.[64]

Lactate Measurement and Interpretation in Equine Neonates

Blood lactate concentrations are higher in normal neonatal foals than normal adult horses for the first 24 to 72 hours of life.[74–76] Reported blood or plasma lactate concentrations (mean $\pm$ SD) measured at or shortly after birth have ranged between 2.38 $\pm$ 1.03 mmol/L[76] and 4.9 $\pm$ 1.0 mmol/L.[74] A recent study reported that mean ($\pm$SD) lactate concentration immediately post partum in 26 healthy foals was 3.8 $\pm$ 1.9 mmol/L (median 3.4 mmol/L, range 1.7–10.2 mmol/L).[75] In that study, lactate concentrations steadily decreased over the first 3 days of life, but median concentration at 72 hours (1.7 mol/L) remained slightly higher than normal adult concentrations and was high ($\leq$3.6 mmol/L) in some apparently normal foals.[75] Blood lactate concentrations in foals aged between 1 and 6 months are the same as concentrations in adults. The cause of the increased lactate concentrations in normal newborn foals is not known for certain but might be related to a combination of peripartum events and immature hepatic function, because fetal lactate concentrations are close to adult values.[77] Lactate is also an important carbohydrate substrate in the fetus, and this might contribute to the normal periparturient hyperlactatemia.[78] This situation complicates slightly the interpretation of blood lactate concentrations measured at a single time point (eg, admission) in equine neonates; however, a steady decrease toward adult concentrations should be seen.[75,79]

Although limited when compared with human medicine, an increasing number of studies have reported significantly higher lactate concentrations at hospital admission in nonsurviving equine neonates when compared with survivors.[59,63,71,75,79,80] Some, but not all, studies have detected significant differences in admission lactate concentrations when foals are categorized on the basis of primary disease.[75,79,80] As would be expected, foals in septic shock or with hypoxic-ischemic (neonatal) encephalopathy generally have higher lactate concentrations at admission when compared with foals with enteritis/colitis or a localized bacterial infection (eg, septic arthritis or an infected umbilical remnant).[76,80,81] The primary diagnosis also seems to have an effect on the clinical significance or usefulness of admission lactate concentration. A prospective study[59] enrolling 643 foals at 13 referral centers found that the risk of nonsurvival increased by 14% for every 1 mmol/L increase in admission blood lactate concentration across the entire population. For major diagnoses of sepsis, unspecified enterocolitis, unspecified colic, trauma, immune-related disease (not including failure of passive transfer of immunity), and respiratory disease, there was a statistically significant increase in the risk of nonsurvival for every 1 mmol/L increase in admission blood lactate concentration.[59] In contrast, increasing admission lactate concentrations were not associated with an increased risk of nonsurvival in foals with a major diagnosis of prematurity/dysmaturity and, perhaps surprisingly, perinatal asphyxia syndrome.[59] The clinical significance of these results is not yet clear, but they might provide an interesting insight into the causes of hyperlactatemia in sick neonatal foals. However, as the investigators of the study note, some caution should be exercised when interpreting their results. The time to presentation might vary considerably between major diagnostic categories and likely has an important effect on admission lactate concentration. Further, despite the size of the study, the number of foals (or the number of nonsurviving foals) in some groups was small, making robust statistical analysis difficult.

As with studies in humans and adult horses, there is considerable overlap between surviving and nonsurviving neonatal foals in the range of blood lactate concentrations measured at admission. Although the sensitivity and specificity of lactate concentration in predicting outcome are typically modest (in the range of 60%–75%), several studies have developed cutoffs that allow prediction of survival with some accuracy. In an earlier study, overall survival to discharge was 67% but was greater than 80% for foals with admission arterial lactate concentrations less than 3.9 mmol/L and decreased to less than 40% for foals with lactate concentrations greater than 6.0 mmol/L.[80] Using an admission lactate concentration of 6.9 mmol/L as a cutoff, outcome was accurately predicted in more than 85% of cases in a general population of sick foals.[79] If a lactate concentration of 3.2 mmol/L was used as a cutoff at 24 hours after admission, outcome could be accurately predicted in 94% of cases.[79]

When measured serially in hospitalized equine neonates, mean blood lactate concentrations are consistently higher in nonsurvivors when compared with survivors.[33,63,80] Furthermore, the OR for survival decreases for every day that lactate concentration remains increased.[63] Not all studies evaluating equine neonates have detected a statistically significant relationship between the rate at which blood lactate concentration decreases and patient outcome.[79,80] However, when changes in lactate concentration over time were used to approximate lactate clearance, the rate of decline in blood lactate concentration was lower in nonsurvivors.[63] A second study enrolling 643 foals has shown that lactate concentrations in surviving foals decreased steadily over the first 48 hours of hospitalization, and by 72 hours after admission, median lactate concentration in survivors was normal (1.3 mmol/L).[71] Although lactate concentration decreased in nonsurviving foals, it did so at a slower rate and remained increased (median 2.1 mmol/L) at 72 hours after admission.[71] The changes in lactate concentration in neonatal foals are opposite to those reported in adult horse, in which the rate of decrease in lactate concentrations was initially higher in nonsurvivors.[29] The reason (or reasons) for the delay in achieving normolactatemia in nonsurviving foals is unknown but might reflect decreased hepatic metabolism, continued reliance on lactate as an energy source, or perhaps an underlying increase in lactate production unrelated to tissue oxygen delivery. The notion that processes other than poor tissue perfusion might be driving hyperlactatemia in critically ill foals is supported by the only modest association between lactate concentration and arterial blood pressure reported in several studies.[63,80] Further, a correlation between lactate concentration and evidence of systemic inflammatory response syndrome has been identified in some studies.[80]

Limitations in the Clinical Use of Blood Lactate Concentrations

Correct interpretation of blood lactate concentrations in critically ill horses requires accurate and precise measurement and knowledge of the appropriate normal reference interval. As already discussed, a range of lactate meters are used in equine practice, but only a few of those have been validated for use in horses. Of those meters that have been evaluated, performance of 1 popular model was poor when whole blood samples were used; performance improved considerably when plasma samples were used, but this obviously limits the field usefulness of these meters.[11] Blood lactate concentration varies with age in normal neonatal foals; however, the reported reference intervals are variable, and it might be sensible to establish center-specific ranges.[75] Ponies and miniature horses with gastrointestinal disease seem to have higher admission blood lactate concentrations when compared with full size horses with similar diseases, and clinicians need to be mindful of this when advising clients on prognosis.[70]

There is typically considerable overlap in the admission blood lactate concentrations of survivors and nonsurvivors in both adult and neonate equine studies. Further, when lactate concentrations are serially measured, the difference between survivors and nonsurvivors after admission is often subtle. In 1 study evaluating adult horses, median L-lactate concentration was statistically significantly higher in nonsurvivors at all time points tested, but the (median) lactate concentration at 12, 24, and 48 hours after admission in nonsurviving horses was within commonly accepted reference limits (<1.5 mmol/L).[29] In that study, median blood lactate concentration at 72 hours after admission in surviving horses was 0.70 mmol/L (range 0.70–2.10 mmol/L) and 1.80 mmol/L (range 0.70–2.60 mmol/L) in nonsurvivors.[29] The subtle changes in lactate concentrations over the course of hospitalization and small differences between surviving and nonsurviving horses highlight the need for accurate and precise measurement. In all studies, there have been surviving animals with high lactate concentrations for the length of the study and some nonsurviving animals with normal lactate concentrations throughout.

Blood lactate concentrations can be a relatively insensitive indicator of tissue perfusion and oxygen delivery. This situation is compounded if inappropriate reference intervals are used. Many texts cite 2.5 mmol/L as the upper end of normal for blood lactate concentrations in adult horses; however, blood lactate concentration in normal adults horses is invariably less than 1.5 mmol/L, and most horses have lactate concentrations less than 1.0 mmol/L. Changes in lactate concentrations were minimal after removal of a substantial volume of blood in 1 experimental study.[81] Median lactate concentration after removal of 16 mL/kg of blood (approximately 8 L for a 500-kg horse) was only 1.35 mmol/L (mean 2.2 ± 1.0 mmol/L), although the response to blood loss by individual hoses was highly variable (range 0.5–6.7 mmol/L).[81] Further, if an animal has time to replenish vascular volume from interstitial or intracellular reserves, blood lactate concentrations might be normal in the face of a clinically relevant fluid deficit.

SUMMARY

The admission lactate concentration of most horses returns to normal ranges fairly rapidly with appropriate therapy, suggesting that decreased tissue perfusion is the most important cause of hyperlactatemia in critically ill horses.[29,72] Because cardiac disease is rare in horses, addressing hypovolemia should be the priority when hyperlactatemia is encountered in horses. However, hyperlactatemia can occur with normal tissue oxygen delivery, and this likely indicates the presence of a severe inflammatory response.[3] Lactate concentrations have been used to evaluate prognosis for almost 40 years in equine (and human) medicine; this alone suggests that the practice has some merit.[65] Serial lactate measurement, measurement of lactate clearances, or other measures reflecting the magnitude and duration of hyperlactatemia might enable more accurate prognostication but might also provide valuable insight into disease pathogenesis in critically ill horses.[25] Serial lactate measurement could be a valuable therapeutic guide, although studies to support this are lacking in equine medicine.

REFERENCES

1. Ewaschuk JB, Naylor JM, Palmer R, et al. D-lactate production and excretion in diarrheic calves. J Vet Intern Med 2004;18:744–7.
2. Gore DC, Jahoor F, Hibbert JM, et al. Lactic acidosis during sepsis is related to increased pyruvate production, not deficits in tissue oxygen availability. Ann Surg 1996;224:97–102.
3. James JH, Luchette FA, McCarter FD, et al. Lactate is an unreliable indicator of tissue hypoxia in injury or sepsis. Lancet 1999;354:505–8.
4. Kline JA, Thornton LR, Lopaschuk GD, et al. Lactate improves cardiac efficiency after hemorrhagic shock. Shock 2000;14:215–21.
5. Schurr A. Lactate: the ultimate cerebral oxidative energy substrate? J Cereb Blood Flow Metab 2006;26:142–52.
6. Cruz RS, de Aguiar RA, Turnes T, et al. Intracellular shuttle: the lactate aerobic metabolism. ScientificWorldJournal 2012;2012:420984.
7. Hashimoto T, Hussien R, Oommen S, et al. Lactate sensitive transcription factor network in L6 cells: activation of MCT1 and mitochondrial biogenesis. FASEB J 2007;21:2602–12.

8. Rasanen LA, Lampinen KJ, Poso AR. Responses of blood and plasma lactate and plasma purine concentrations to maximal exercise and their relation to performance in standardbred trotters. Am J Vet Res 1995;56:1651–6.

9. Rainger JE, Evans DL, Hodgson DR, et al. Distribution of lactate in plasma and erythrocytes during and after exercise in horses. Br Vet J 1995;151:299–310.

10. Ewaschuk JB, Naylor JM, Barabash WA, et al. High-performance liquid chromatographic assay of lactic, pyruvic and acetic acids and lactic acid stereoisomers in calf feces, rumen fluid and urine. J Chromatogr B Analyt Technol Biomed Life Sci 2004;805:347–51.

11. Tennent-Brown BS, Wilkins PA, Lindborg S, et al. Assessment of a point-of-care lactate monitor in emergency admissions of adult horses to a referral hospital. J Vet Intern Med 2007;21:1090–8.

12. Williamson CC, James EA, James MP, et al. Horse plasma lactate determinations: comparison of wet and dry chemistry methods and the effect of storage. Equine Vet J 1996;28:406–8.

13. Lindner A. Measurement of plasma lactate concentration with Accusport. Equine Vet J 1996;28:403–5.

14. Evans DL, Golland LC. Accuracy of Accusport for measurement of lactate concentrations in equine blood and plasma. Equine Vet J 1996;28:398–402.

15. Saulez MN, Cebra CK, Dailey M. Comparative biochemical analyses of venous blood and peritoneal fluid from horses with colic using a portable analyser and an in-house analyser. Vet Rec 2005;157:217–23.

16. Sloet van Oldruitenborgh-Oosterbaan MM, van den Broek ET, Spierenburg AJ. Evaluation of the usefulness of the portable device Lactate Pro for measurement of lactate concentrations in equine whole blood. J Vet Diagn Invest 2008;20:83–5.

17. Hollis AR, Dallap Schaer BL, Boston RC, et al. Comparison of the Accu-Chek Aviva point-of-care glucometer with blood gas and laboratory methods of analysis of glucose measurement in equine emergency patients. J Vet Intern Med 2008;22:1189–95.

18. Tennent-Brown BS, Koenig A, Williamson LH, et al. Comparison of three point-of-care blood glucose meters for use in adult and juvenile alpacas. J Am Vet Med Assoc 2011;239:380–6.

19. Allen SE, Holm JE. Lactate: physiology and clinical utility. J Vet Emerg Crit Care 2008;18:123–32.

20. Pang DS, Boysen S. Lactate in veterinary critical care: pathophysiology and management. J Am Anim Hosp Assoc 2007;43:270–9.

21. Ferrante PL, Kronfeld DS. Effect of sample handling on measurement of plasma glucose and blood lactate concentrations in horses before and after exercise. Am J Vet Res 1994;55:1497–500.

22. Robergs RA, Ghiasvand F, Parker D. Biochemistry of exercise-induced metabolic acidosis. Am J Physiol Regul Integr Comp Physiol 2004;287:R502–16.

23. Kreisberg RA. Glucose-lactate inter-relations in man. N Engl J Med 1972;287:132–7.

24. Connor H, Woods HF, Ledingham JG, et al. A model of L(+)-lactate metabolism in normal man. Ann Nutr Metab 1982;26:254–63.

25. De Pedro P, Wilkins PA, McMichael MA, et al. Exogenous L-lactate clearance in adult horses. J Vet Emerg Crit Care (San Antonio) 2012;22:564–72.

26. Bellomo R. Bench-to-bedside review: lactate and the kidney. Crit Care 2002;6:322–6.

27. Fall PJ, Szerlip HM. Lactic acidosis: from sour milk to septic shock. J Intensive Care Med 2005;20:255–71.
28. Lagutchik MS, Ogilvie GK, Wingfield WE, et al. Lactate kinetics in veterinary critical care: a review. J Vet Emerg Crit Care 1996;6:81–95.
29. Tennent-Brown BS, Wilkins PA, Lindborg S, et al. Sequential plasma lactate concentrations as prognostic indicators in adult equine emergencies. J Vet Intern Med 2010;24:198–205.
30. McCarter FD, James JH, Luchette FA, et al. Adrenergic blockade reduces skeletal muscle glycolysis and Na(+), K(+)-ATPase activity during hemorrhage. J Surg Res 2001;99:235–44.
31. Vary TC. Increased pyruvate dehydrogenase kinase activity in response to sepsis. Am J Physiol 1991;260:E669–74.
32. Vary TC, Siegel JH, Nakatani T, et al. Effect of sepsis on activity of pyruvate dehydrogenase complex in skeletal muscle and liver. Am J Physiol 1986;250: E634–40.
33. Stacpoole PW, Wright EC, Baumgartner TG, et al. A controlled clinical trial of dichloroacetate for treatment of lactic acidosis in adults. The Dichloroacetate-Lactic Acidosis Study Group. N Engl J Med 1992;327:1564–9.
34. Stacpoole PW, Nagaraja NV, Hutson AD. Efficacy of dichloroacetate as a lactate-lowering drug. J Clin Pharmacol 2003;43:683–91.
35. Haji-Michael PG, Ladriere L, Sener A, et al. Leukocyte glycolysis and lactate output in animal sepsis and ex vivo human blood. Metabolism 1999;48:779–85.
36. Parry BW, Anderson GA, Gay CC. Prognosis in equine colic: a comparative study of variables used to assess individual cases. Equine Vet J 1983;15:211–5.
37. Latson KM, Nieto JE, Beldomenico PM, et al. Evaluation of peritoneal fluid lactate as a marker of intestinal ischaemia in equine colic. Equine Vet J 2005; 37:342–6.
38. Chrusch C, Bands C, Bose D, et al. Impaired hepatic extraction and increased splanchnic production contribute to lactic acidosis in canine sepsis. Am J Respir Crit Care Med 2000;161:517–26.
39. Levraut J, Ciebiera JP, Chave S, et al. Mild hyperlactatemia in stable septic patients is due to impaired lactate clearance rather than overproduction. Am J Respir Crit Care Med 1998;157:1021–6.
40. Severin PN, Uhing MR, Beno DW, et al. Endotoxin-induced hyperlactatemia results from decreased lactate clearance in hemodynamically stable rats. Crit Care Med 2002;30:2509–14.
41. Revelly JP, Tappy L, Martinez A, et al. Lactate and glucose metabolism in severe sepsis and cardiogenic shock. Crit Care Med 2005;33:2235–40.
42. Douzinas EE, Tsidemiadou PD, Pitaridis MT, et al. The regional production of cytokines and lactate in sepsis-related multiple organ failure. Am J Respir Crit Care Med 1997;155:53–9.
43. Cairns CB, Moore FA, Haenel JB, et al. Evidence for early supply independent mitochondrial dysfunction in patients developing multiple organ failure after trauma. J Trauma 1997;42:532–6.
44. Chiolero R, Revelly JP, Tappy L. Energy metabolism in sepsis and injury. Nutrition 1997;13:45S–51S.
45. Parker MG, Fraser GL, Watson DM, et al. Removal of propylene glycol and correction of increased osmolar gap by hemodialysis in a patient on high dose lorazepam infusion therapy. Intensive Care Med 2002;28:81–4.
46. Levy B. Bench-to-bedside review: is there a place for epinephrine in septic shock? Crit Care 2005;9:561–5.

47. Luft FC. Lactic acidosis update for critical care clinicians. J Am Soc Nephrol 2001;12(Suppl 17):S15–9.

48. Nielsen HB, Bredmose PP, Stromstad M, et al. Bicarbonate attenuates arterial desaturation during maximal exercise in humans. J Appl Physiol (1985) 2002; 93:724–31.

49. Manohar M, Goetz TE, Hassan AS. NaHCO(3) does not affect arterial O(2) tension but attenuates desaturation of hemoglobin in maximally exercising thoroughbreds. J Appl Physiol (1985) 2004;96:1349–56.

50. Sillos EM, Shenep JL, Burghen GA, et al. Lactic acidosis: a metabolic complication of hematologic malignancies: case report and review of the literature. Cancer 2001;92:2237–46.

51. Elfenbein J, Credille B, Camus M, et al. Hypoglycemia and hyperlactatemia associated with lymphoma in an Angus cow. J Vet Intern Med 2008;22:1441–3.

52. James JH, Wagner KR, King JK, et al. Stimulation of both aerobic glycolysis and Na(+)-K(+)-ATPase activity in skeletal muscle by epinephrine or amylin. Am J Physiol 1999;277:E176–86.

53. James JH, Fang CH, Schrantz SJ, et al. Linkage of aerobic glycolysis to sodium-potassium transport in rat skeletal muscle. Implications for increased muscle lactate production in sepsis. J Clin Invest 1996;98:2388–97.

54. Vary TC. Sepsis-induced alterations in pyruvate dehydrogenase complex activity in rat skeletal muscle: effects on plasma lactate. Shock 1996;6:89–94.

55. Kellum JA, Kramer DJ, Lee K, et al. Release of lactate by the lung in acute lung injury. Chest 1997;111:1301–5.

56. De Backer D, Creteur J, Zhang H, et al. Lactate production by the lungs in acute lung injury. Am J Respir Crit Care Med 1997;156:1099–104.

57. De Backer D, Creteur J, Silva E, et al. The hepatosplanchnic area is not a common source of lactate in patients with severe sepsis. Crit Care Med 2001;29: 256–61.

58. Grosche A, Morton AJ, Graham AS, et al. Effect of large colon ischemia and reperfusion on concentrations of calprotectin and other clinicopathologic variables in jugular and colonic venous blood in horses. Am J Vet Res 2013;74: 1281–90.

59. Borchers A, Wilkins PA, Marsh PM, et al. Association of admission L-lactate concentration in hospitalised equine neonates with presenting complaint, periparturient events, clinical diagnosis and outcome: a prospective multicentre study. Equine Vet J Suppl 2012;(41):57–63.

60. Nguyen HB, Rivers EP, Knoblich BP, et al. Early lactate clearance is associated with improved outcome in severe sepsis and septic shock. Crit Care Med 2004; 32:1637–42.

61. Bakker J, Gris P, Coffernils M, et al. Serial blood lactate levels can predict the development of multiple organ failure following septic shock. Am J Surg 1996; 171:221–6.

62. McNelis J, Marini CP, Jurkiewicz A, et al. Prolonged lactate clearance is associated with increased mortality in the surgical intensive care unit. Am J Surg 2001; 182:481–5.

63. Wotman K, Wilkins PA, Palmer JE, et al. Association of blood lactate concentration and outcome in foals. J Vet Intern Med 2009;23:598–605.

64. Hashimoto-Hill S, Magdesian KG, Kass PH. Serial measurement of lactate concentration in horses with acute colitis. J Vet Intern Med 2011;25:1414–9.

65. Moore JN, Owen RR, Lumsden JH. Clinical evaluation of blood lactate levels in equine colic. Equine Vet J 1976;8:49–54.

66. Orsini JA, Elser AH, Galligan DT, et al. Prognostic index for acute abdominal crisis (colic) in horses. Am J Vet Res 1988;49:1969–71.
67. Furr MO, Lessard P, White NA 2nd. Development of a colic severity score for predicting the outcome of equine colic. Vet Surg 1995;24:97–101.
68. Parry BW, Gay CC, Anderson GA. Assessment of the necessity for surgical intervention in cases of equine colic: a retrospective study. Equine Vet J 1983;15: 216–21.
69. Parry BW, Anderson GA, Gay CC. Prognosis in equine colic: a study of individual variables used in case assessment. Equine Vet J 1983;15:337–44.
70. Dunkel B, Kapff JE, Naylor RJ, et al. Blood lactate concentrations in ponies and miniature horses with gastrointestinal disease. Equine Vet J 2013;45:666–70.
71. Borchers A, Wilkins PA, Marsh PM, et al. Sequential L-lactate concentration in hospitalised equine neonates: a prospective multicentre study. Equine Vet J 2013;45:2–7.
72. Radcliffe RM, Divers TJ, Fletcher DJ, et al. Evaluation of L-lactate and cardiac troponin I in horses undergoing emergency abdominal surgery. J Vet Emerg Crit Care (San Antonio) 2012;22:313–9.
73. Johnston K, Holcombe SJ, Hauptman JG. Plasma lactate as a predictor of colonic viability and survival after 360 degrees volvulus of the ascending colon in horses. Vet Surg 2007;36:563–7.
74. Kitchen H, Rossdale PD. Metabolic profiles of newborn foals. J Reprod Fertil Suppl 1975;(23):705–7.
75. Castagnetti C, Pirrone A, Mariella J, et al. Venous blood lactate evaluation in equine neonatal intensive care. Theriogenology 2010;73:343–57.
76. Magdesian GK. Blood lactate levels in neonatal foals: normal values and temporal effects in the post-partum period. International Veterinary Emergency and Critical Care Symposium. New Orleans (LA), September, 2003. p. 174.
77. Fowden AL, Taylor PM, White KL, et al. Ontogenic and nutritionally induced changes in fetal metabolism in the horse. J Physiol 2000;528(Pt 1):209–19.
78. Pere MC. Materno-foetal exchanges and utilisation of nutrients by the foetus: comparison between species. Reprod Nutr Dev 2003;43:1–15.
79. Henderson IS, Franklin RP, Wilkins PA, et al. Association of hyperlactatemia with age, diagnosis, and survival in equine neonates. J Vet Emerg Crit Care 2008;18: 496–502.
80. Corley KT, Donaldson LL, Furr MO. Arterial lactate concentration, hospital survival, sepsis and SIRS in critically ill neonatal foals. Equine Vet J 2005;37:53–9.
81. Magdesian KG, Fielding CL, Rhodes DM, et al. Changes in central venous pressure and blood lactate concentration in response to acute blood loss in horses. J Am Vet Med Assoc 2006;229:1458–62.

Crystalloid and Colloid Therapy

Langdon Fielding, DVM*

KEYWORDS

- Intravenous fluids • Colloids • Crystalloids • Hyperchloremia • Fluid overload
- Edema

KEY POINTS

- Hyperchloremia should be avoided because of an association with morbidity and possibly mortality.
- A chloride-restrictive intravenous fluid strategy may help to prevent hyperchloremia.
- Modifications to the classic understanding of the Starling equation question the use of intravenous colloids.
- The evidence supporting the use of intravenous colloids is more limited after the retraction of numerous clinical studies that indicated a benefit for intravenous colloid administration.
- Fluid overload–associated morbidity is increasingly recognized and should be avoided.

In all areas of medicine new research findings modify current recommendations and standards of practice. In intravenous fluid therapy, there are 3 new developments that equine practitioners should consider as they make clinical decisions:

1. Avoiding hyperchloremia: the negative effects of hyperchloremia continue to be investigated, but increasing evidence suggests that fluid therapy plans that are chloride restrictive may be advantageous compared with a chloride-liberal plan.
2. Avoiding colloids: modifications to understanding of the Starling equation have changed the model for transcapillary fluid movement and questioned the theoretic efficacy of colloids. In addition, significant studies supporting colloid use have been retracted in major journals. Equine clinicians should carefully consider whether the remaining evidence supports the use of colloids in equine practice.
3. Avoiding fluid overload: there is increasing evidence that morbidity and mortality are affected by fluid overload and that more attention should be paid to avoidance of this problem.

The author has nothing to disclose and no conflicts of interest.
Loomis Basin Equine Medical Center, 2973 Penryn Road, Penryn, CA 95663, USA
* Private practice.
E-mail address: langdonfielding@yahoo.com

These 3 issues are considered in detail in this article. Following this discussion, these modifications are incorporated into a standard fluid therapy plan that can be used for equine practice.

HYPERCHLOREMIA

A few key observations have raised awareness about the possible negative effects of hyperchloremia. Taken together, these observations suggest that a chloride-restrictive strategy may be appropriate for intravenous fluid therapy.[1] To summarize a few of the main findings:

1. Hyperchloremia has been identified as a predictor of mortality in multiple studies.[2] In addition to mortality, the increased serum chloride is often associated with other negative prognostic indicators.[3,4]
2. Randomized clinical trials comparing high-chloride and low-chloride fluids suggest a more normal electrolyte and acid-base profile of patients in the low-chloride groups.[5] In addition, the more chloride-restrictive strategies have a lower incidence of acute kidney injury.[1]
3. There are experimental benefits of intravenous fluids with lower chloride concentrations compared with fluids with higher chloride concentrations. The benefits primarily include increased renal perfusion with fluids that have a lower chloride concentration and a decrease in the concentration of inflammatory cytokines.[6-9]

In order to avoid hyperchloremia in critical patients, 2 factors must be considered for clinical equine practice. (1) Can intravenous fluids that are lower in chloride be used in place of higher chloride fluids? (2) Is there a problem with the excretion of chloride in critical patients that needs to be considered? These two questions are considered here.

In equine practice, most patients are resuscitated with an isotonic crystalloid solution and the 3 commonly available solutions are 0.9% saline, lactated Ringer solution, and Plasma-Lyte A (or Normosol R). The electrolyte (sodium, potassium, and chloride) concentrations of these fluids are listed in **Table 1**. Plasma-Lyte A has the lowest chloride concentration and saline (0.9%) has the highest (significantly greater than equine plasma). Although specific metabolic derangements (hypochloremic metabolic alkalosis) may warrant the use of 0.9% saline, a general recommendation for Normosol R as a first choice for resuscitation of hypovolemia in horses is likely to be appropriate.

Avoiding intravenous fluids that are high in chloride helps to decrease the amount of administered chloride, but serum chloride may still increase if the kidney is retaining the ion. One recent study concluded that the urinary excretion of chloride may play a bigger role in the development of hyperchloremia than the type of intravenous fluid administered.[10] More research is needed in this area but, if sick patients retain chloride inappropriately, new therapeutic options may be possible. The development of hyperchloremia is likely to be a combination of increased input through intravenous fluid therapy and an abnormal retention of chloride through the kidney.

Table 1
Sodium, potassium, and chloride concentrations of 3 common isotonic resuscitation fluids used in horses

	Lactated Ringer	Normal Saline	Plasma-Lyte A/Normosol R
Sodium (mEq/L)	130	154	140
Potassium (mEq/L)	4	0	5
Chloride (mEq/L)	109	154	98

COLLOID RESEARCH REVISITED

Recommendations for the use of colloids as an intravenous resuscitation fluid have been based on a traditional understanding of the Starling equation. By increasing the oncotic pressure of the plasma volume, these fluids were thought to help pull fluid out of the interstitium and expand the intravascular space. Combined with the positive results from clinical trials, colloid administration became a standard part of many equine practices. However, 2 recent developments have undermined these recommendations for colloid use:

1. The no-absorption rule has been proposed as one of many modifications to understanding of the Starling equation and transcapillary fluid movement.[11]
2. Several clinical studies published by Joachim Boldt that had been a significant component of the support for colloid use in practice have recently been retracted.[12] In addition to these retractions, some smaller reviews of colloids have been criticized because of the investigators' relationship with the commercial production of these fluids.[13]

These two new findings deserve more explanation, but taken together they may have shifted the balance of support away from the use of colloids in most clinical cases.

The No-Absorption Rule

The no-absorption rule indicates that fluid cannot be absorbed from the interstitium back into the vascular space (**Fig. 1**). It relies on a new understanding of transcapillary fluid dynamics that goes beyond the Starling equation.[14]
   The Starling equation is often given as:

$$\text{Net filtration} = K_f\,[(P_{cap} - P_{int}) - (\pi_{plasma} - \pi_{int})]$$

The term K_f represents the permeability of the capillary wall. The term P_{cap} refers to the hydrostatic pressure within the vascular space. The term P_{int} refers to the hydrostatic pressure within the interstitial space. The term π_{plasma} represents plasma oncotic pressure and is described earlier. The term π_{int} refers to the oncotic pressure generated by the proteins and mucopolysaccharides within the interstitium.

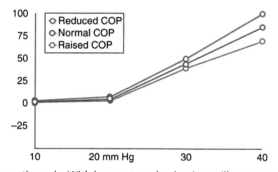

Fig. 1. The no-absorption rule. With less-acute reduction in capillary pressure, the glycocalyx model preserves filtration at a very low rate without a phase of absorption, the no-absorption rule. The inflection on the filtration curve is called the J point. COP, capillary osmotic pressure (mm Hg). (*From* Woodcock TE, Woodcock TM. Revised Starling equation and the glycocalyx model of transvascular fluid exchange: an improved paradigm for prescribing intravenous fluid therapy. Br J Anaesth 2012;108:390; with permission.)

Modifications to the Starling equation have included a better understanding of the importance of the hydrostatic pressure (P_{int}) within the interstitial space. Inflammation and other disease states can modify the interstitial space and create a negative pressure that helps to pull fluid into the interstitial space. Changes to the structure of this space may allow it to accumulate fluid.[14] Improving plasma oncotic pressure does not improve the interstitial hydrostatic pressure or prevent fluid accumulation in this space.

In addition, the endothelial glycocalyx layer (EGL) has been described as a space located between the plasma volume and the endothelial cells lining the capillaries (**Fig. 2**).[11,14] The EGL acts as a zone that modifies the interaction of the plasma volume and interstitial space. This zone affects the movement of fluid out of the capillaries and contributes to the no-absorption rule, which suggests that fluid is unlikely ever to move from the interstitium back into the capillaries. Administering a hyperoncotic fluid (such as a synthetic colloid) is unlikely to cause a significant decrease in interstitial fluid volume or have a clinical effect on edema formation.

There are some excellent reviews of transcapillary fluid movement that incorporate many of the newer findings and modifications to the Starling equation.[11,14] Taken together, these findings have caused some investigators to question the rationale for the use of intravenous colloids. However, as more research on this topic becomes available, further recommendations will be made.

Retraction of Studies Supporting Colloid Use

Several clinical studies published by Joachim Boldt have recently been retracted.[12] Some of these studies had supported the use of colloids and were incorporated into larger meta-analyses. Once these studies are removed, the balance of evidence shifts away from any strong support of colloid use.

In addition, the conclusions of some smaller reviews of colloid use have been called into question. These reviews tended to support the use of colloids, but there is concern that the investigators of these reviews may have a financial relationship to companies associated with these colloids.[13] If these smaller reviews are excluded, the remaining studies do not offer any strong support for the use of colloids in clinical practice.

Remaining Evidence Addressing Colloid Use

The recently published CRISTAL trial was a large, multicenter, randomized clinical trial that evaluated fluid resuscitation with crystalloids versus colloids in critically ill patients

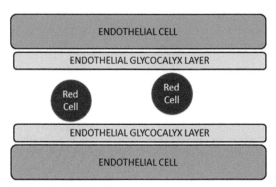

Fig. 2. The EGL and the endothelial cell.

with hypovolemic shock.[15] The study did not find a significant difference between the fluid protocols (crystalloid vs colloid) in 28-day mortality; however, they did note an improvement in 90-day mortality in the colloid group. The clinical significance of this finding at 90 days is unclear.

Other recent studies and reviews have primarily acknowledged the increased risk of acute kidney injury (AKI) with colloids and/or found an increased risk of mortality.[16–19] One recent large review in humans concluded that "The current evidence suggests that all [hydroxyethyl starches] increase the risk in [acute kidney injury] and [renal replacement therapy] in all patient populations."[20] Although studies evaluating the association between AKI and hydroxyethyl starches in horses are lacking, it is logical that these products would have similar effects in horses.

It is possible that certain subgroups may still benefit from colloid administration, but more research is needed. The conclusion by many of these investigators is that the evidence no longer supports the use of colloids, especially given the increased expense of these solutions. Many of the negative effects of colloids have not been shown in horses, but appropriately sized clinical trials have not been completed.

FLUID OVERLOAD

Intravenous fluid therapy has long been considered a cornerstone of emergency medicine in all species. Although much of the focus in the last decade has been on an aggressive initial resuscitation protocol,[21] recent studies have raised concerns about the negative effects of fluid overload.[22] One particular study was a large, randomized clinical trial that was halted before completion because of the increased mortality in the more aggressive fluid resuscitation group.[23] This study has been criticized for the lack of monitoring (central venous pressure, blood pressure, and so forth) during aggressive fluid resuscitation; however, this is a common scenario in many equine practices. It is clear that there are potential negative effects of large volume fluid resuscitation in some groups of patients (**Box 1**).

Some investigators have raised concerns that the warning signs of fluid overload are not being appropriately recognized.[24] This lack of recognition contributes to fluid-associated morbidity.[24] Further education about the recognition of fluid overload may help to mitigate some of these effects.

Risk factors for fluid overload are listed in **Box 2**. In horses, AKI associated with diminished urine production is probably the most common risk factor for fluid overload. Any horse with evidence of AKI (50% increase in baseline creatinine; urine production <1 mL/kg/h despite adequate fluid resuscitation) should be monitored carefully for fluid overload to prevent the morbidity and mortality associated with this condition.

Early recognition of fluid overload requires careful attention and monitoring by the attending clinician. Although visual evidence of dependent edema is easy to identify,

---

Box 1
Negative associations with fluid overload

1. Mortality[27–29]

2. Slower intestinal healing[30]

3. Delayed wound healing[31]

4. Ileus[32]

5. Pulmonary dysfunction

Box 2
Risk factors for the development of fluid overload

1. Hypoproteinemia
2. Renal failure
3. Heart failure
4. Blood product administration

---

earlier and more subtle signs can be missed. Clinical and laboratory parameters that can be used to recognize fluid overload are listed in **Table 2**.

More important than recognizing the clinical signs of fluid overload, monitoring fluid balance provides an early alert that fluid overload is imminent. There are 2 basic approaches to fluid balance monitoring:

1. Body weight changes. Twice-daily body weight measurements can indicate fluid retention or fluid loss over a given time period. However, baseline data are often unknown and it can be challenging to determine whether weight gain is the gradual restoration of normovolemia or the gradual accumulation of excess fluid volume.
2. Calculation of ins and outs. A daily summary of fluid losses and fluid gains can determine whether overall daily fluid balance is positive or negative. In an intensive care unit setting, fluid losses are typically urinary or gastrointestinal (reflux and/or diarrhea). Less commonly, fluid loss into the thoracic or abdominal cavity (particularly if being removed through drainage) should be considered. Fluid gains are typically oral or intravenous.

If possible, both methods (body weight changes and in/out calculations) should be used and compared along with clinical examination and laboratory data. However, in a recent study, the calculation of ins and outs was the most effective means for recognizing fluid retention.[25] In practical terms, if a scale is not readily available then monitoring changes in body weight is not possible. Measurement of ins and outs requires a urinary catheter and collection system, but even monitoring the fluids administered and the amounts of reflux obtained over time can help illuminate trends in losses and gains.

Treatment of Fluid Overload

The treatment of fluid overload consists of 2 main components: (1) decreased fluid administration; and (2) increased fluid removal.

Decreasing the rate of fluid administration is a simple step that can restore a more normal fluid balance. Choosing a new rate of fluid administration can be challenging depending on requirements because of ongoing disease. Temporary reduction of the

---

Table 2
Recognition of fluid overload

Clinical examination	Edema: ventral abdomen, legs, head Adventitial lung sounds Serial body weight increases (after rehydration)
Hemodynamic monitoring	Central venous pressure
Pulmonary function impairment	Partial pressure arterial oxygen

rate by 50% is often a good compromise, with reassessment after 4 to 6 hours. If severe signs of overload are evident, fluids should be stopped until fluid has been removed.

Increasing fluid removal or excretion is a major part of the treatment of fluid overload. The administration of intravenous furosemide is warranted in critical cases of fluid overload because this often leads to a rapid increase in fluid loss. In cases of anuric renal failure, furosemide administration may not improve kidney function, but increased urine production may allow better fluid management. Furosemide can be given as a bolus dose (1–2 mg/kg, intravenously) or as a continuous infusion (0.12 mg/kg/h following a 0.12-mg/kg loading dose, intravenously). In cases of anuria, renal replacement therapies are a newer option for fluid removal, but this therapy has only limited availability.[26]

In summary, fluid overload is increasingly recognized as a cause of morbidity and mortality in critical care. Prevention of fluid overload is best achieved by recognizing the risk factors and the use of judicious rates of fluid administration. If fluid overload occurs, treatment should include decreased administration and the administration of furosemide.

THE BASIC COMPONENTS OF A FLUID THERAPY PLAN

The 4 main aspects of all fluid therapy plans are based on 4 key questions:

1. Are intravenous fluids indicated?
2. What type of fluid is most appropriate?
3. What rate of fluid administration is needed?
4. When can fluids be stopped?

Are Intravenous Fluids Indicated?

Indications for the initiation of intravenous fluid therapy are generally broad. At a minimum, they have included any horse with signs of hypovolemia/hypoperfusion including:

1. Tachycardia
2. Poor pulse quality
3. Prolonged capillary refill time (>2 seconds)
4. Pale mucous membranes
5. Cold extremities
6. Decreased mentation
7. Decreased urine output (<0.5–1.0 mL/kg/h)
8. Poor jugular refill

Other tests that may support a finding of hypovolemia/hypoperfusion include:

1. Increased blood lactate concentration (>2.0 mmol/L)
2. Decreased central venous oxygen saturation
3. Negative central venous pressure
4. Decreased mean arterial pressure (<60 mm Hg)

Although an abnormality in a single parameter does not necessarily warrant intravenous fluids, multiple abnormal findings should prompt the clinician to begin fluid therapy. Many clinicians also initiate intravenous fluid therapy for horses that may be at risk for developing hypovolemia even if clinical signs are not yet present. A typical example might be a horse with fevers that is not drinking or eating and is likely to become dehydrated and hypovolemic if the illness persists.

In addition to horses with hypovolemia, intravenous fluids are often started in patients with ongoing renal disease, ongoing gastrointestinal disease (ie, feed impactions), and as protection against renal injury from nephrotoxic agents (oxytetracycline, aminoglycosides, nonsteroidal antiinflammatory drugs, and so forth). The criteria for initiating intravenous fluid therapy in this group of horses are often less well defined. They frequently depend on the clinician's assessment of the risks and benefits of therapy.

Type of Fluid

The type of intravenous fluid chosen for treatment is one of the most active areas of research in fluid therapy in humans, horses, and other species. Equine clinicians are often faced with practical choices and must choose the type of fluids to stock on a truck (or in a hospital) long before the needs of a specific case are known. However, the new information described earlier suggests that the choices may have become simpler.

Initial Resuscitation Fluid

As a general recommendation, the initial resuscitation fluid for most clinical cases of hypovolemia is an isotonic crystalloid that approximately reflects the normal electrolyte concentrations of horses. Avoidance of hyperchloremia should also be considered because of the possible negative effects, which suggests that Plasma-Lyte A (Normosol R) is likely the best choice for most cases because of its concentration of sodium and chloride. Fluids that have electrolyte concentrations that are subtly different from normal plasma concentrations may result in derangements over extended periods of administration, particularly if the horse is not drinking water or if renal function is compromised.

Based on the discussions earlier, high-chloride fluids (0.9% saline and possibly even lactated Ringer solution) may not be as appropriate as a low-chloride fluid such as Normosol R or Plasma-Lyte A. In addition, there is no evidence that colloid administration offers any benefits compared with crystalloids and may increase the risk for AKI in humans. Plasma-Lyte A likely represents the safest fluid choice for resuscitation, particularly in the absence of clinical laboratory testing to guide fluid choice.

Rate of Fluid Administration

A protocol of fluid resuscitation that incorporates small bolus administration followed by reassessment is a safe and practical approach in emergency equine medicine. A 20-mL/kg bolus of Plasma-Lyte A is typically administered over 30 to 60 minutes followed by reassessment of the perfusion parameters listed earlier. The bolus doses can be repeated until the perfusion parameters normalize or until early signs of fluid overload develop.

Once the resuscitation phase has ended, most adult horses can be changed to a rate of 2 to 4 mL/kg/h of an isotonic crystalloid. Based on the new concerns of fluid overload associated morbidity, this postresuscitation phase may now be more conservative and a lower rate (even 1–3 mL/kg/h) may be appropriate as long as urine production is maintained (>1 mL/kg/h) and signs of hypovolemia do not return.

End Points to Fluid Administration

Given the research described earlier, fluid overload should be recognized early and avoided. If the patient is not producing urine (>0.5–1 mL/kg/h) despite adequate volume replacement, fluid bolus administration should be stopped and a more careful assessment of renal function should be completed (blood work, urinalysis, ultrasonography of bladder and kidneys). If other signs of fluid overload develop (edema, respiratory dysfunction), fluid administration should be stopped and furosemide should be considered.

In conclusion, intravenous fluid therapy in equine practice should continue to evolve based on research and recommendations in other species. Although large, randomized studies in horses are lacking, equine critical care can benefit from observations in human medicine. The changes described in this article are anticipated to improve morbidity and even mortality in horses based on the findings in other species.

REFERENCES

1. Yunos N, Bellomo R, Hegarty C, et al. Association between a chloride-liberal vs chloride-restrictive intravenous fluid administration strategy and kidney injury in critically ill adults. JAMA 2012;308:1566–72.
2. Boniatti MM, Cardoso PR, Castilho RK, et al. Is hyperchloremia associated with mortality in critically ill patients? A prospective cohort study. J Crit Care 2011; 26:175–9.
3. Noritomi DT, Soriano FG, Kellum JA, et al. Metabolic acidosis in patients with severe sepsis and septic shock: a longitudinal quantitative study. Crit Care Med 2009;37:2733–9.
4. Silva Junior JM, Neves EF, Santana TC, et al. The importance of intraoperative hyperchloremia. Rev Bras Anestesiol 2009;59:304–13.
5. Young JB, Utter GH, Schermer CR, et al. Saline versus plasma-lyte A in initial resuscitation of trauma patients: a randomized trial. Ann Surg 2014;259(2): 255–62.
6. Kellum JA, Song M, Venkataraman R. Effects of hyperchloremic acidosis on arterial pressure and circulating inflammatory molecules in experimental sepsis. Chest 2004;125:243–8.
7. Aksu U, Bezemer R, Yavuz B, et al. Balanced vs unbalanced crystalloid resuscitation in a near-fatal model of hemorrhagic shock and the effects on renal oxygenation, oxidative stress, and inflammation. Resuscitation 2012;83:767–73.
8. Chowdhury AH, Cox EF, Francis ST, et al. A Randomized, controlled, double-blind crossover study on the effects of 1-L infusions of 6% hydroxyethyl starch suspended in 0.9% saline (Voluven) and a balanced solution (Plasma Volume Redibag) on blood volume, renal blood flow velocity, and renal cortical tissue perfusion in healthy volunteers. Ann Surg 2014;259(5):881–7.
9. Chowdhury AH, Cox EF, Francis ST, et al. A randomized, controlled, double-blind crossover study on the effects of 2-L infusions of 0.9% saline and plasma-lyte 148 on renal blood flow velocity and renal cortical tissue perfusion in healthy volunteers. Ann Surg 2012;256:18–24.
10. Masevicius FD, Vazquez AR, Enrico C, et al. Urinary strong ion difference is a major determinant of plasma chloride concentration changes in postoperative patients. Rev Bras Ter Intensiva 2013;25:197–204.
11. Woodcock TE, Woodcock TM. Revised Starling equation and the glycocalyx model of transvascular fluid exchange: an improved paradigm for prescribing intravenous fluid therapy. Br J Anaesth 2012;108:384–94.
12. Reilly C. Retraction. Notice of formal retraction of articles by Dr Joachim Boldt. Br J Anaesth 2011;107:116–7.

13. Hartog CS, Skupin H, Natanson C, et al. Systematic analysis of hydroxyethyl starch (HES) reviews: proliferation of low-quality reviews overwhelms the results of well-performed meta-analyses. Intensive Care Med 2012;38:1258–71.

14. Levick JR, Michel CC. Microvascular fluid exchange and the revised Starling principle. Cardiovasc Res 2010;87:198–210.

15. Annane D, Siami S, Jaber S, et al, CRISTAL Investigators. Effects of fluid resuscitation with colloids vs crystalloids on mortality in critically ill patients presenting with hypovolemic shock: the CRISTAL randomized trial. JAMA 2013;310:1809–17.

16. Serpa Neto A, Veelo DP, Peireira VG, et al. Fluid resuscitation with hydroxyethyl starches in patients with sepsis is associated with an increased incidence of acute kidney injury and use of renal replacement therapy: a systematic review and meta-analysis of the literature. J Crit Care 2014;29(1):185.e1–7.

17. Perel P, Roberts I, Ker K. Colloids versus crystalloids for fluid resuscitation in critically ill patients. Cochrane Database Syst Rev 2013;(2):CD000567.

18. Patel A, Waheed U, Brett SJ. Randomised trials of 6% tetrastarch (hydroxyethyl starch 130/0.4 or 0.42) for severe sepsis reporting mortality: systematic review and meta-analysis. Intensive Care Med 2013;39:811–22.

19. Zarychanski R, Abou-Setta AM, Turgeon AF, et al. Association of hydroxyethyl starch administration with mortality and acute kidney injury in critically ill patients requiring volume resuscitation: a systematic review and meta-analysis. JAMA 2013;309:678–88.

20. Mutter TC, Ruth CA, Dart AB. Hydroxyethyl starch (HES) versus other fluid therapies: effects on kidney function. Cochrane Database Syst Rev 2013;(7):CD007594.

21. Rivers E, Nguyen B, Havstad S, et al, Early Goal-Directed Therapy Collaborative Group. Early goal-directed therapy in the treatment of severe sepsis and septic shock. N Engl J Med 2001;345:1368–77.

22. Godin M, Bouchard J, Mehta RL. Fluid balance in patients with acute kidney injury: emerging concepts. Nephron Clin Pract 2013;123:238–45.

23. Maitland K, Kiguli S, Opoka RO, et al. Mortality after fluid bolus in African children with severe infection. N Engl J Med 2011;364:2483–95.

24. Walsh SR, Walsh CJ. Intravenous fluid-associated morbidity in postoperative patients. Ann R Coll Surg Engl 2005;87:126–30.

25. Schneider AG, Baldwin I, Freitag E, et al. Estimation of fluid status changes in critically ill patients: fluid balance chart or electronic bed weight? J Crit Care 2012;27:745.e7–12.

26. Wong DM, Witty D, Alcott CJ, et al. Renal replacement therapy in healthy adult horses. J Vet Intern Med 2013;27(2):308–16.

27. Askenazi DJ, Koralkar R, Hundley HE, et al. Fluid overload and mortality are associated with acute kidney injury in sick near-term/term neonate. Pediatr Nephrol 2013;28:661–6.

28. Vaara ST, Korhonen AM, Kaukonen KM, et al, The FINNAKI study group. Fluid overload is associated with an increased risk for 90-day mortality in critically ill patients with renal replacement therapy: data from the prospective FINNAKI study. Crit Care 2012;16:R197.

29. Payen D, de Pont AC, Sakr Y, et al, Sepsis Occurrence in Acutely Ill Patients (SOAP) investigators. A positive fluid balance is associated with a worse outcome in patients with acute renal failure. Crit Care 2008;16:R74.

30. Kulemann B, Timme S, Seifert G, et al. Intraoperative crystalloid overload leads to substantial inflammatory infiltration of intestinal anastomoses–a histomorphological analysis. Surgery 2013;154:596–603.

31. Huang Q, Zhao R, Yue C, et al. Fluid volume overload negatively influences delayed primary facial closure in open abdomen management. J Surg Res 2014; 187(1):122–7.
32. Lobo DN, Bostock KA, Neal KR, et al. Effect of salt and water balance on recovery of gastrointestinal function after elective colonic resection: a randomised controlled trial. Lancet 2002;359:1812–8.

Acute Hemorrhage and Blood Transfusions in Horses

Margaret C. Mudge, VMD

KEYWORDS

- Equine • Blood • Transfusion • Hemorrhage • Hemostasis

KEY POINTS

- Acute hemorrhage can be life-threatening and may require blood transfusion, especially if greater than 25% blood loss has occurred.
- A variety of topical hemostatic agents and techniques can be used to control external hemorrhage.
- Initial transfusions may be performed without crossmatch in an emergency, and blood recipients should be monitored closely for any transfusion reactions.
- Ideally transfuse with fresh whole blood to replace 25% to 50% of the blood lost.
- Cell salvage devices can also be used to collect autologous blood in cases of intracavitary and intraoperative blood loss.

INTRODUCTION

Acute hemorrhage in horses can result in severe shock, and even when treated can be fatal. The principles of treating hemorrhagic shock have been described in the human and veterinary literature.[1,2] Adjunctive methods of controlling hemorrhage, such as newer hemostatic devices and products on the market, have potential for use in the horse. In addition, recently published information about blood storage and transfusion in human, canine, and equine medicine may help guide blood transfusion procedures. Acute hemorrhage in the horse does present some unique challenges because of the volume of hemorrhage and difficult access to sources of the bleeding.

ACUTE HEMORRHAGE
Recognizing Acute Hemorrhage in the Horse

Acute hemorrhage can be external, such as arterial lacerations or epistaxis, or internal, such as splenic lacerations or uterine artery bleeding. Blood loss requiring transfusion

The author has nothing to disclose.
Department of Veterinary Clinical Sciences, The Ohio State University, 601 Vernon L. Tharp Street, Columbus, OH 43210, USA
E-mail address: Margaret.Mudge@cvm.osu.edu

has been reported with gastrointestinal, urogenital, and sinonasal surgeries.[3–5] Internal hemorrhage may be more difficult to diagnose because of the absence of visible blood loss. Abdominal ultrasound and abdominocentesis can indentify hemoperitoneum, although the underlying cause is not always evident.

For internal and external hemorrhage, it is critical to recognize the signs of hemorrhagic shock, which include tachycardia, tachypnea, cold extremities, anxiety or depression, pale mucous membranes, and prolonged capillary refill time. Horses with hemoperitoneum may also demonstrate colic and abdominal distension.[6] Clinicopathologic findings often include hyperlactatemia, hypoproteinemia, and anemia. However, the packed cell volume (PCV) and total protein (TP) may be normal in horses with acute whole blood loss. Splenic contraction can maintain PCV in the acute stages of hemorrhage, and PCV and TP remain normal until fluid redistributes from the interstitial spaces (over the first 12 hours if intravenous fluids are not administered). Serial monitoring of PCV and TP is recommended, and emergency resuscitation and transfusion may be indicated based on clinical signs rather than a specific PCV value.

Physiologic Hemostasis and Medical Management

After initial trauma, vasoconstriction occurs initially, followed by platelet activation, adhesion, and aggregation. Disruption of the endothelium exposes tissue factor-bearing cells, leading to activation of clotting factors and production of thrombin. The activated platelet serves as a congregation site for coagulation factors, and ultimately a stable fibrin clot is formed. Coagulopathy is rarely the cause of acute hemorrhage in horses, and further diagnostics and specific treatments are needed if coagulopathy is suspected (see article on coagulopathies elsewhere in this issue).

Stabilization with intravenous fluids has the potential to worsen bleeding, although specific medications can be used to enhance clot stability. Intravenous fluids are needed to restore intravascular volume in cases of hemorrhagic shock. Unfortunately, these fluids can also dilute platelets and clotting factors and negatively affect clot formation. In vitro and in vivo studies have demonstrated the hypocoagulatory effect of hydroxyethyl starch in humans and horses.[7–9] Large volumes of fluid may also raise blood pressure and disrupt the clot; therefore, conservative fluid resuscitation is recommended over shock doses of intravenous fluids, at least until definitive surgical hemostasis can be achieved. Human trauma and animal model studies demonstrate the benefits of delayed or hypotensive resuscitation.[10,11] Prolonged hypotension has deleterious effects, and therefore a balance must be achieved between treating hypotension and stabilizing the clot.

In addition to blood products (discussed later), medications can be used to promote hemostasis. Synthetic lysine analogues, epsilon aminocaproic acid, and tranexamic acid act through reversibly blocking the lysine binding sites of plasminogen, thus inhibiting fibrinolysis. Aminocaproic acid was administered in 92% of mares with periparturient hemorrhage in a recent study.[12] Some mares in this retrospective study received 10% formalin, conjugated estrogens, and yunnan baiyao as adjunctive hemostatic treatments. Intravenous formaldehyde is thought to potentiate hemostasis through activating platelets or endothelium. However, infusion of formaldehyde in normal horses did not result in any change in hemostatic variables.[13] Naloxone has also been advocated for use during uncontrolled hemorrhage. Naloxone may lessen hypotension through counteracting the endogenous opiate vasodilation and bradycardia that can occur with severe acute hemorrhage.[14,15]

Surgical and Topical Hemostasis

Ideally definitive surgical hemostasis may be achieved with ligatures, stapling devices, or electrothermal vessel sealing devices (LigaSure, Covidien, Mansfield, MA, USA). For bleeding from a distal limb, a tourniquet can be applied to achieve immediate reduction in blood loss. This step should not be overlooked and should be performed before fluid resuscitation. If a bandage is already in place, a pneumatic or Esmarch tourniquet and suture material for ligatures should be available before the bandage is removed. For external areas on which a tourniquet cannot be applied, manual pressure should be used.

Diffuse capillary bleeding, especially from parenchymal organs, can be difficult to control. Topical hemostatic agents may be useful to control internal hemorrhage (during surgery) or nasal hemorrhage (**Table 1**). Mechanical hemostatic agents, such as purified gelatin sponge (Gelfoam, Pfizer, New York, NY, USA) and oxidized regenerated cellulose (Surgicel, Ethicon, Somerville, NJ, USA), are useful in small areas of uncontrolled capillary bleeding. Vascular sealants include fibrin glues (Tisseel, Baxter, Deerfield, IL), thrombin-gelatin matrix (FloSeal, Baxter, Deerfield, IL, USA), and polyethylene glycol (PEG) polymer (Coseal, Baxter, Deerfield, IL, USA).

The following are recommendations for an approach to acute hemorrhage in the horse:

- Provide bleeding control with compression or tourniquet, if possible
- Administer delayed or hypotensive resuscitation until ready for definitive treatment
- Maintain mean arterial pressure at approximately 60 mm Hg
- Administer 20 mL/kg of intravenous bolus of crystalloid fluid; alternatively, 2 to 4 mL/kg of intravenous hypertonic saline may be given if immediate volume resuscitation is needed
- Prepare for blood transfusion if estimate greater than 30% blood loss

Hemorrhage from guttural pouch mycosis presents a unique challenge because the site of the bleed (internal carotid, external carotid or maxillary artery) is inaccessible and because the bleed can be rapidly fatal. Experimental studies show that ligation of the ipsilateral common carotid artery (CCA) will actually increase blood flow through the internal carotid artery from retrograde flow via the circle of Willis.[16] Therefore, temporary ligation of both CCAs is recommended to slow the bleeding and allow a clot to form.

Table 1
Topical hemostats

Type of Hemostat	Examples	Indications	Side Effects/Comments
Mechanical	Gelfoam, Surgicel	Control capillary and small venous/arterial bleeding	May interfere with skin healing; potential for embolization
Biologic: thrombin	FloSeal, Surgiflo	Adjunct to hemostasis	May interfere with skin healing; potential for embolization
Fibrin sealants	Tisseel, Evicel	Used in human cardiopulmonary bypass procedures	Potential for embolization; possible hypersensitivity reactions
Sealants: polyethylene glycol polymers	Coseal	Mechanical seal for leaking areas	Expensive

BLOOD TRANSFUSION
Criteria for Transfusion

Practitioners must often decide whether to give a blood transfusion. This decision is more difficult when the bleeding is internal and acute, and the PCV remains within the normal range.

The following are indications for blood transfusion in cases of acute hemorrhage:

- Estimated blood loss greater than 30% (**Table 2**)
- PCV less than 20% during an acute bleeding episode
- Blood lactate level of 4 mmol/L or more after fluid therapy
- Oxygen extraction ratio 50% or greater

Transfusion guidelines or "triggers" described in the human medical literature include liberal hemoglobin triggers of 10 g/dL and restrictive triggers of 7 g/dL. The more restrictive strategy seems to reduce morbidity and in-hospital mortality.[17] Similar studies have not been performed in horses. Conditions such as pulmonary or cardiovascular disease may increase the transfusion trigger, because the patient has less ability to compensate for the anemia. The need for transfusion may be more difficult to assess in a horse under anesthesia, because the heart rate often remains stable despite severe blood loss. In the anesthetized horse, mucous membrane color, capillary refill time, blood pressure, and oxygenation are the parameters that should be monitored.[18]

Blood Products

Fresh whole blood is the blood product most commonly used to replenish red blood cell mass in horses. Blood transfusion is not a common procedure even in the largest referral centers; therefore, it is more practical to collect blood from donor horses on an as-needed basis rather than store large volumes of blood. Stored packed red blood cells are commonly used in human medicine; however, recent studies indicate the negative effects of stored blood. Red blood cells are known to undergo changes in pH, glucose, ATP, and osmotic stability during storage, known as the "storage lesion." Authors of a meta-analysis of studies examining the effect of blood storage duration on mortality in humans concluded that transfusion with older stored blood significantly increases the risk of death.[19] Prestorage leukoreduction has been shown to decrease the inflammatory response to transfusion in dogs, and has also been shown to reduce microparticle formation.[20,21]

Table 2
Acute hemorrhage: estimated blood loss

% Blood Loss	Heart Rate	Respiratory Rate	Capillary Refill Time	Blood Pressure	Other Physical Examination Findings
<15	Normal	Normal	Normal	Normal	Possible mild anxiety
15–30	Increased	Increased	Mildly prolonged	Normal	Mild anxiety
30–40	Moderate to severely increased	Increased	Prolonged	Decreased	Anxious or depressed; cool extremities
>40	Severely increased	Increased	Very pale mucous membranes	Severe hypotension	Obtunded; cool extremities

No reports compare the inflammatory or mortality effects of stored blood in the horse, but based on information in other species, fresh blood would be ideal when available. The red blood cell (RBC) half-life of 24-hour-old allogeneic equine whole blood is approximately 20 days, compared with a 45-day half-life for 24-hour-old autologous equine blood.[22,23] Other advantages of fresh whole blood include viable platelets and coagulation factors in plasma.

Packed RBCs are indicated for horses with chronic anemia or those with acute blood loss and normovolemia, such as when volume has been replaced by crystalloid fluids. In most cases of acute hemorrhage, whole blood is the appropriate blood product. When packed RBCs are needed, stored blood may be used or blood may be processed into plasma and RBC components. In the field, whole blood may be allowed to sediment, with only the RBC-rich component given if volume overload is a concern. If packed RBCs are used for massive transfusions during acute hemorrhage, additional fresh frozen plasma and platelet concentrate should also be transfused.

Oxyglobin (OPK Biotech, Cambridge, MA, USA) is hemoglobin-based oxygen carrying solution that is an alternative treatment for anemia when blood is not available. Oxyglobin has been used in horses, although it is currently not available in the United States.[24,25]

Plasma transfusions are not useful for restoring oxygen-carrying capacity, but may be used as an adjunctive treatment when colloid and clotting factors are desired. Fresh and fresh frozen plasma contain immunoglobulins and coagulation factors II, V, VII, VIII, IX, X, XI, and XII and antithrombin and proteins C and S.

Blood Donors and Pretransfusion Testing

The ideal equine blood donor is a healthy, large (>500 kg), well-behaved gelding. No true universal donor exists, because there are 8 equine blood groups and 30 different factors. Donors should ideally be negative for the Aa and Qa alloantigens, because these are most commonly associated with hemolytic reactions. Donors should not have alloantibodies to any blood groups. Several equine blood-typing laboratories are available (**Box 1**).

When a blood-typed donor is not available, a healthy gelding may be used for the first transfusion. Horses that have had foals or previous transfusions are at a higher risk of carrying RBC antibodies, and therefore are not suitable donors. These horses are also at a higher risk of experiencing adverse reactions when they receive a blood transfusion. Donkeys and mules have an RBC antigen known as *donkey factor*, and therefore should not be used as blood donors for horses, and should not receive horse blood unless it is confirmed to be free of anti–donkey factor antibody.

A crossmatch may not be necessary in emergency situations when the recipient has had no prior exposure to blood products. Horses can develop alloantibodies within 1 week of transfusion, and therefore a crossmatch is recommended before a second transfusion is performed.[26] The major crossmatch detects reactions between the donor's RBCs and the recipient's serum. The minor crossmatch detects reactions between the recipient's RBCs and the donor's serum. Routine crossmatching evaluates hemagglutination; however, the more common hemolytic reactions are not detected unless rabbit complement is added to the reaction mixture. Although stored donor samples can be used for convenience, fresh blood samples yield more reproducible results in crossmatching.[27]

Blood Collection and Storage

Up to 20% of the donor horse's blood volume can be collected at one time. Blood volume is estimated as 8% of body weight; therefore, a 500 kg horse can donate up to 8 L

Box 1
Equine blood typing laboratories

Central Laboratory Receiving

Room 1033, Veterinary Medical Teaching Hospital

One Garrod Drive

University of California, Davis

Davis, CA 95616

Phone: 530-752-8684

http://www.vetmed.ucdavis.edu/vmth/small_animal/laboratory/local-assets/pdfs/UC_Davis_VMTH_EQUINE_BLOOD_TYPING-NI_Submission_Form.pdf

University of Kentucky

Animal Genetic Testing & Research Laboratory

108 Gluck Equine Research Center

Lexington, KY 40546-0000

Phone: 859-218-1212

http://www2.ca.uky.edu/gluck/AGTRL.asp

Rood and Riddle Veterinary Laboratory

2150 Georgetown Road

Lexington, KY 40511

Phone: 859-233-0331

http://www.roodandriddle.com/laboratory.html

Hagyard Equine Medical Institute

4250 Iron Works Pike

Lexington, KY 40511-8412

Phone: 859-259-3685

http://www.hagyard.com/Hagyard-Laboratory.html

---

of blood. Crystalloid fluids can be given to replace blood volume, and are recommended when greater than 15% blood volume is collected. A short length (1 or 2 inches), large diameter (10–14 gauge) intravenous catheter is placed in the jugular vein, and blood flow can be improved by directing the catheter toward the head (opposite venous flow) and putting pressure on the jugular veins below the catheter. Blood flow is further improved through using vacuum suction. Although vacuum suction into glass bottles results in inactivation of platelets and damage to red blood cells, vacuum suction into blood bags has been shown to result in good-quality blood product.[28]

When blood is collected for immediate transfusion, a simple anticoagulant solution such as 3.2% sodium citrate is adequate. When blood is going to be stored, a pH buffer and source of glucose are needed. Citrate-phosphate-dextrose with adenine (CPDA-1, Fenwal Inc., Lake Zurich, IL, USA) is available in bags for collection of 450 mL of blood. Using fresh whole blood has many advantages, including improved RBC viability, lower lactate and potassium levels, and fewer inflammatory reactions. However, it is not always practical to use an on-site donor or to give all the blood at one time. Additionally, autologous blood may be stored for some high-risk elective surgical procedures. Autologous equine blood stored in CPDA-1 for 28 days had a half-life of 29 days, whereas compatible allogeneic equine blood stored for only 24 hours has a 20-day half-life.[22,23] When blood is collected for storage, special attention should be given to sterility, and leukoreduction should be considered before storage. Blood should be stored in a dedicated blood bank refrigerator at 4°C.

Transfusion Volume and Technique

The amount of blood required for transfusion can be estimated from the amount of blood lost during acute hemorrhage (see **Table 2**) or through using the desired PCV in cases of more chronic anemia. The equation in **Box 2** may be used if the horse's PCV accurately reflects the blood loss.

The entire blood volume lost does not need to be replaced, because volume has already increased through mobilization of interstitial fluid, voluntary intake of water, and administration of intravenous fluids. Approximately 25% to 50% of blood lost should be replaced, and packed RBCs may be used if concern exists about volume overload. The volume to be transfused may be limited by the volume of blood that can be safely removed from the donor horse. Blood should be delivered using an inline filter to remove any blood clots or fibrin.

Adverse Effects

Blood products should be given slowly for the first 15 minutes to monitor the horse for any signs of acute transfusion reaction. The reported incidence of blood transfusion reactions in horses is 16%.[3] Crossmatches do not accurately predict transfusion reactions, and therefore horses should be monitored closely even when a compatible crossmatch is confirmed. Acute hemolytic reactions typically occur when there are preexisting RBC antibodies. Severe hemolysis has also been reported in dogs after administration of improperly stored hemolyzed blood.[29] Clinical signs include hemoglobinemia, hemoglobinuria, and systemic inflammatory response. The transfusion should be stopped immediately when an acute hemolytic reaction is suspected. Delayed hemolytic transfusion reactions can occur more than 24 hours after transfusion and result in similar clinical signs of hemolysis.

Other potential transfusion reactions include fever and allergic reaction. Type I hypersensitivity reactions can manifest as urticaria, pruritis, piloerection, and, in severe cases, anaphylactic shock. Mild to moderate reactions may be treated with an antihistamine or corticosteroid. Severe reactions require treatment with epinephrine (0.01–0.02 mL/kg intravenously of a 1:1000 solution). Inflammatory reactions such as fever are more likely to occur with older stored units of blood. Transfusion-associated

---

Box 2
Blood transfusion equation

Blood transfusion volume (mL) = body weight (kg) × 80 mL/kg × [(desired PCV − actual PCV)/donor PCV]

Example: One day after an acute episode of hemorrhage, a 500-kg horse has a PCV of 15% and is pale and tachycardic. If a PCV of 25% is desired and the donor horse has a PCV of 38%, the horse will require approximately 10 L of whole blood.

500 kg × 80 mL/kg × [(25−15)/38] = 10,526 mL = 10.5 L

immunomodulation and transfusion-related acute lung injury have been recognized in human and canine patients but have not been described in horses.[30,31]

Adverse effects seem to be less common with plasma transfusions than with blood transfusions. For commercial equine plasma, an incidence of 8.7% in foals and 0% in adults was reported, and a 10.0% incidence was reported for noncommercial equine plasma.[32,33]

Other potential negative effects of transfusion include infectious disease transmission, bacterial contamination, citrate toxicity, and circulatory overload. Serum hepatitis has been reported with commercial plasma transfusion in horses.[34] Another possible negative effect is sensitization of the broodmare to other blood groups, leading to neonatal isoerythrolysis in subsequent foals.

Alternative Sources of Blood

Situations may occur in which donor horses are not readily available or a compatible donor cannot be found. Autologous transfusion is a good alternative in these cases, and may be preferable in some situations because the RBC half-life is longer and the incidence of transfusion reaction should be minimal. When moderate to severe hemorrhage is anticipated with a planned surgical procedure, preoperative autologous donation may be used. Similar to preoperative blood donation procedures in human medicine, blood is collected from the equine patient 2 to 3 weeks before surgery and is stored in CPDA-1 or a similar storage medium in a blood bank refrigerator. This blood is then transfused during surgery or after surgery, if needed.

Autologous cell salvage is a technique that can be used with acute cavitary or intraoperative hemorrhage. Cell salvage systems collect blood into a reservoir, anticoagulate and filter the blood, and then wash and resuspend the RBCs in preparation for delivery through a leukoreduction filter. In the past, cell salvage was not recommended in cases of neoplasia or bacterial contamination. Recent human studies have demonstrated the safety of cell salvage in these situations.[35] The successful use of a blood salvage device has been reported in dogs undergoing cardiotomy and hemoperitoneum surgeries.[36] Cavitary blood from the abdomen or thorax may be collected without the use of a cell salvage device and may be administered with routine blood filtration sets if contamination is not suspected.[4] Anticoagulation is still recommended; however, less volume of anticoagulant can be used, because cavitary blood is defibrinated.

SUMMARY

Blood transfusions are not commonly needed in horses, but the practitioner should be prepared to collect and transfuse blood when needed for acute hemorrhage. The goal of the transfusion is to improve oxygen delivery to the tissues, and therefore transfusion should be used along with other fluid resuscitation and any surgical stabilization. The common practice of transfusing fresh whole blood from donor horses is the most appropriate treatment for severe acute hemorrhage. Adjunctive treatment with topical hemostats and antifibrinolytics can also be useful when managing cases of acute hemorrhage.

REFERENCES

1. Dutton RP. Haemostatic resuscitation. Br J Anaesth 2012;109(Suppl 1):i39–46.
2. Rudloff E, Kirby R. Fluid resuscitation and the trauma patient. Vet Clin North Am Small Anim Pract 2008;38(3):645–52.

3. Hurcombe SD, Mudge MC, Hinchcliff KW. Clinical and clinicopathologic variables in adult horses receiving blood transfusions: 31 cases (1999-2005). J Am Vet Med Assoc 2007;231:267–74.

4. Waguespack R, Belknap J, Williams A. Laparoscopic management of postcastration haemorrhage. Equine Vet J 2001;33:510–3.

5. Nickels FA. Nasal passages and paranasal sinuses. In: Auer JA, Stick JA, editors. Equine surgery. St Louis (MO): Elsevier; 2012. p. 557–68.

6. Pusterla N, Fecteau ME, Madigan JE, et al. Acute hemoperitoneum in horses: a review of 19 cases (1992-2003). J Vet Intern Med 2005;19(3):344–7.

7. Hartog CS, Reuter D, Loesche W, et al. Influence of hydroxyethyl starch (HES) 130/0.4 on hemostasis as measured by viscoelastic device analysis: a systematic review. Intensive Care Med 2011;37(11):1725–37.

8. Jones PA, Tomasic M, Gentry PA. Oncotic, hemodilational, and hemostatic effects of isotonic saline and hydroxyethyl starch solutions in clinically normal ponies. Am J Vet Res 1997;58(5):541–8.

9. Blong AE, Epstein KL, Brainard BM. In vitro effects of three formulations of hydroxyethyl starch solutions on coagulation and platelet function in horses. Am J Vet Res 2013;74:712–20.

10. Bickell WH, Bruttig SP, Millnamow MA, et al. The detrimental effects of intravenous crystalloid after aortotomy in swine. Surgery 1991;110:529–36.

11. Bickell WH, Wall MJ, Pepe PE, et al. Immediate versus delayed fluid resuscitation for hypotensive patients with penetrating torso injuries. N Engl J Med 1994; 331(17):1105–9.

12. Arnold CE, Payne M, Thompson JA, et al. Periparturient hemorrhage in mares: 73 cases (1998-2005). J Am Vet Med Assoc 2008;232:1345–51.

13. Taylor EL, Sellon DC, Wardrop KJ, et al. Effects of intravenous administration of formaldehyde on platelet and coagulation variables in healthy horses. Am J Vet Res 2000;61:1191–6.

14. Weld JM, Kamerling SG, Combie JD, et al. The effects of naloxone on endotoxic and hemorrhagic shock in horses. Res Commun Chem Pathol Pharmacol 1984; 44:227–38.

15. Ludbrook J, Rutter PC. Effect of naloxone on haemodynamic responses to acute blood loss in unanaesthetized rabbits. J Physiol 1988;400:1–14.

16. Woodie JB, Ducharme NG, Gleed RD, et al. In horses with guttural pouch mycosis or after stylohyoid bone resection, what arterial ligation(s) could be effective in emergency treatment of hemorrhagic crisis. Vet Surg 2002;31: 498–9.

17. Salpeter SR, Buckley JS, Chatterjee S. Impact of more restrictive blood transfusion strategies on clinical outcomes: a meta-analysis and systematic review. Am J Med 2014;127(2):124–31.e3.

18. Wilson DV, Rondenay Y, Shance PU. The cardiopulmonary effects of severe blood loss in anesthetized horses. Vet Anaesth Analg 2003;30:81–7.

19. Wang D, Sun J, Solomon SB, et al. Transfusion of older stored blood and risk of death: a meta-analysis. Transfusion 2012;52(6):1184–95.

20. McMichael MA, Smith SA, Galligan A, et al. Effect of leukoreduction on transfusion-induced inflammation in dogs. J Vet Intern Med 2010;24:1131–7.

21. Herring JM, Smith SA, McMichael MA, et al. Microparticles in stored canine RBC concentrates. Vet Clin Pathol 2013;42(2):163–9.

22. Owens SD, Johns JL, Walker NJ. Use of an in vitro biotinylation technique for determination of posttransfusion survival of fresh and stored autologous red blood cells in Thoroughbreds. Am J Vet Res 2010;71(8):960–6.

23. Mudge MC, Borjesson DL, Walker NJ, et al. Post-transfusion survival of biotin-labeled allogeneic RBCs in adult horses. Vet Clin Pathol 2012;41(1):56–62.

24. Belgrave RL, Hines MT, Keegan RD, et al. Effects of a polymerized ultrapurified bovine hemoglobin blood substitute administered to ponies with normovolemic anemia. J Vet Intern Med 2002;16:396–403.

25. Maxson AD, Giger U, Sweeney CR, et al. Use of bovine hemoglobin preparation in the treatment of cyclic ovarian hemorrhage in a miniature horse. J Am Vet Med Assoc 1993;203:1308–11.

26. Wong PL, Nickel LS, Bowling AT, et al. Clinical survey of antibodies against red blood cells in horses after homologous blood transfusion. Am J Vet Res 1986; 47:2566–71.

27. Harris M, Nolen-Walston R, Ashton W, et al. Effect of sample storage on blood crossmatching in horses. J Vet Intern Med 2012;26(3):662–7.

28. Conversy B, Blais MC, Carioto L, et al. Comparison of gravity collection versus suction collection for transfusion purposes in dogs. J Am Anim Hosp Assoc 2013;49:301–7.

29. Patterson J, Rousseau A, Kessler RJ, et al. In vitro lysis and acute transfusion reactions with hemolysis caused by inappropriate storage of canine red blood cell products. J Vet Intern Med 2011;25:927–33.

30. Prittie JE. Controversies related to red blood cell transfusion in critically ill patients. J Vet Emerg Crit Care (San Antonio) 2010;20(2):167–76.

31. Thomovsky EJ, Bach J. Incidence of acute lung injury in dogs receiving transfusions. J Am Vet Med Assoc 2014;244(2):170–4.

32. Hardefeldt LY, Keuler N, Peek SF. Incidence of transfusion reactions to commercial equine plasma. J Vet Emerg Crit Care (San Antonio) 2010;20(4):421–5.

33. Wilson EM, Holcombe SJ, Lamar A, et al. Incidence of transfusion reactions and retention of procoagulant and anticoagulant factor activities in equine plasma. J Vet Intern Med 2009;23(2):323–8.

34. Aleman M, Nieto JE, Carlson GP. Serum hepatitis associated with commercial plasma transfusion in horses. J Vet Intern Med 2005;19:120–2.

35. Ashworth A, Klein AA. Cell salvage as a part of a blood conservation strategy in anaesthesia. Br J Anaesth 2010;105(4):401–16.

36. Kellett-Gregory LM, Seth M, Adamantos S, et al. Autologous canine red blood cell transfusion using cell salvage devices. J Vet Emerg Crit Care (San Antonio) 2013; 23(1):82–6.

Coagulopathies in Horses

Kira L. Epstein, DVM

KEYWORDS

- Hypocoagulation • Hypercoagulation • Hypofibrinolysis • Hyperfibrinolysis • DIC

KEY POINTS

- Normal hemostasis has 3 components: primary hemostasis (formation of platelet plug), secondary hemostasis (formation of meshwork of cross-linked fibrin), and fibrinolysis (breakdown of cross-linked fibrin).
- Excessive bleeding is commonly caused by hypocoagulation, but it can also be caused by hyperfibrinolysis or increased anticoagulant activity. Excessive thrombosis is caused by the opposite changes.
- Clinical signs and coagulation panel (platelet count, prothrombin time [PT], activated partial thromboplastin time [aPTT], fibrinogen, antithrombin [AT], and fibrin/fibrinogen degradation products [FDPs]/D-dimers) results can be used for diagnosis and/or directing further testing for coagulopathy.
- If excessive bleeding or thrombosis occurs, specific therapies are available. Any underlying disease and/or predisposing factors including treatments and toxins must be addressed.

INTRODUCTION
Nature of the Problem

When an area of the body is injured or infected, formation of clots or thrombi within the vessels surrounding the area limits blood loss or spread of infection. Just as important as the formation of the clot is limiting the spread of the thrombus to healthy tissue. A balance between coagulant, anticoagulant, fibrinolytic, and antifibrinolytic activities is required for coordinated clot formation and removal. Dysfunction of the coagulation and/or fibrinolytic systems can result in excessive bleeding or thrombosis, depending on the relative imbalance.

Definitions

Normal hemostasis
Normal hemostasis has 3 main components: primary hemostasis, secondary hemostasis, and fibrinolysis (**Box 1**). Although it is convenient to view the process as 3

Disclosures: The author has nothing to disclose.
Department of Large Animal Medicine, College of Veterinary Medicine, University of Georgia, 501 DW Brooks Dr, Athens, GA 30602, USA
E-mail address: kirae@uga.edu

Vet Clin Equine 30 (2014) 437–452
http://dx.doi.org/10.1016/j.cveq.2014.04.002
0749-0739/14/$ – see front matter

> **Box 1**
> **Components of normal hemostasis**
>
> • Primary hemostasis is the formation of a platelet plug.
> • Secondary hemostasis is the formation of a meshwork of cross-linked fibrin that solidifies the platelet plug.
> • Fibrinolysis is the breakdown of cross-linked fibrin.

separate steps, as our understanding improves, it is becoming increasingly clear that the steps are inextricably linked and proceed concurrently. This is a result of the roles of local and circulating cells, including platelets, fibroblasts, endothelial cells, and monocytes.

Primary hemostasis involves the adhesion, activation, and aggregation of platelets. Adhesion occurs when injury to endothelial cells triggers the expression of P-selectin, which can bind to exposed subendothelial collagen, laminin, or fibronectin and released von Willebrand factor (vWF).[1] Platelets are activated by exposure to collagen; products released by other activated platelets, such as thromboxane A_2 (TxA_2), serotonin (5-hydroxytryptamine), and adenosine diphosphate (ADP); or, most potently, thrombin, a product of secondary hemostasis.[2] Activation of the platelet results in release of products from platelet granules to activate and stimulate aggregation of other platelets and provide a localized source of soluble clotting factors and calcium for secondary hemostasis. Activated platelets also synthesize platelet activating factor and TxA_2, change shape and form interplatelet bridges, and express proteins that bind vWF and fibrinogen. One of the most important roles of activated platelets is providing a surface (phospholipid) for and catalyzing the enzymatic reactions of secondary hemostasis.[3] The thrombin, TxA_2, vWF, and ADP in the region then stimulate aggregation.[4]

Healthy endothelial cells limit the expansion of the platelet plug by maintaining a negatively charged surface to repel negatively charged platelets, producing nitric oxide and prostacyclin to inhibit platelet adhesion, activation, and aggregation and cause vasodilation, and producing thrombomodulin and heparans to degrade thrombin and ADPases to degrade ADP.[5]

Secondary hemostasis involves a series of enzymatic reactions with circulating and localized soluble clotting factors (FI-XIII) that ultimately lead to the production of thrombin, which cleaves fibrinogen to fibrin, which is cross-linked by FXIIIa to form a fibrin meshwork. The traditional, cascade, model for secondary hemostasis has 2 convergent pathways that are initiated separately (**Box 2**).

Although the cascade model is useful for understanding coagulation testing, it is now clear that most secondary hemostasis occurs on the surface of cells and is better explained by a cell-based model. The cell-based model has 3 steps: initiation,

> **Box 2**
> **Cascade model of secondary hemostasis**
>
> • The intrinsic and extrinsic pathways activate the common pathway.
> • The intrinsic pathway is stimulated by contact with exposed collagen and involves FXII, FXI, FIX, and FVIII.
> • The extrinsic pathway starts with exposure of tissue factor (TF or FIII) and involves FVII.
> • The common pathway includes FX, FV, and FII.

amplification, and propagation. During initiation, tissue factor (TF) expressed on exposed extravascular fibroblasts or inflamed endothelial cells or monocytes binds to circulating FVIIa. The TF-FVIIa complex on the surface of the cell then activates FX and FIX. The small amount of FXa generates a small amount of thrombin to participate in amplification before it is rapidly inactivated. The FIXa generated can leave the surface and move to the surface of a platelet to participate in propagation. During amplification, the small amount of thrombin generated during initiation activates platelets, cleaves vWF-FVIII complexes, and activates FV, FVIII, and FXI. The activated factors (FVa, FVIIIa, and FXIa) are localized on the activated platelet surface. During propagation, FIXa generated during initiation and from interaction with FXIa on the platelet surface combines with FVIIIa on the platelet surface to generate FXa, which interacts with FVa on the platelet surface to create a large burst of thrombin production.[6]

Secondary hemostasis is limited by several circulating and localized anticoagulants. The most important circulating anticoagulant is AT, which can inactivate FXa, FIIa, FVIIa, FIXa, FXIa, and FXIIa.[7] Heparans located on surrounding healthy endothelium potentiate the activity of AT.[5] Thrombomodulin, also located on the endothelium, binds thrombin, which promotes the inactivation of thrombin, inhibits fibrinogen clotting, platelet and endothelial cell activation, and FV activation, and activates protein C (PC). Activated PC binds to protein S and inactivates FVa and FVIIIa.[8] Another important anticoagulant is tissue factor pathway inhibitor, which inactivates the TF-FVIIa complex and FXa.[9]

Fibrinolysis begins with the activation of plasminogen by tissue plasminogen activator (tPA) released from injured or fibrin-stimulated endothelial cells. tPA cleaves plasminogen to create plasmin. Plasmin cleaves fibrin, thereby degrading clots. The main inhibitors of fibrinolysis are plasminogen activator inhibitor-1, α2-antiplasmin, and thrombin-activatable fibrinolysis inhibitor.

Coagulopathy

Coagulopathy, or abnormal hemostasis, can be caused by increases (hyper-) or decreases (hypo-) in coagulation (primary or secondary hemostasis) or fibrinolysis. Clinically, coagulopathies are separated into those resulting in excessive bleeding (**Box 3**) or thrombosis (**Box 4**).

Disseminated intravascular coagulation (DIC) is an important coagulopathy that can affect horses. DIC typically occurs secondary to systemic diseases that trigger a severe local or systemic inflammatory response. Resulting damage to the endothelium and promotion of coagulation leads to microvascular thrombi formation, ischemia, and possible multiorgan dysfunction. As coagulation proceeds, coagulant, anticoagulant, fibrinolytic, and antifibrinolytic components are consumed, which can result in excessive bleeding.[13] Studies have shown 32% of horses with colitis[14] and 70% of horses with large colon volvulus[15] have clinicopathologic evidence of DIC. In addition,

---

Box 3
Excessive bleeding

- Excessive bleeding is most frequently caused by hypocoagulation but can also be caused by hyperfibrinolysis or increased anticoagulant activity.

- Hypocoagulation can be caused by decreased amount or function of components of primary or secondary hemostasis.

- Hyperfibrinolysis has been proposed to contribute to increased bleeding in several disease states, including trauma[10] and postpartum hemorrhage.[11]

- Increased anticoagulant activity can occur iatrogenically.

Box 4
Excessive thrombosis

- Excessive thrombosis can be caused by hypercoagulation, hypofibrinolysis, or decreased anticoagulant activity.
- It is rare to encounter excessive thrombosis as a primary condition in horses.
- Inflammation causes a variety of changes that promote both primary and secondary hemostasis and inhibit fibrinolysis and anticoagulant activity.[12]

---

approximately 40% of horses[16] with ischemic and inflammatory gastrointestinal disease and 70% of septic foals[17] have histologic and immunohistochemistry findings of fibrin deposits consistent with capillary microthrombi and DIC on postmortem examination.

CLINICAL FINDINGS
Physical Examination

Excessive bleeding

In theory, the most likely clinical signs of hypocoagulation vary depending on whether primary or secondary hemostasis is affected. When primary hemostasis is affected, bleeding from mucosal surfaces and bleeding, bruising, ecchymoses, and hematoma formation secondary to traumatic or iatrogenic (eg, surgical, venipuncture, and catheter) wounds are most common. In cases of thrombocytopenia, but not thrombocytopathia, petechiae are also often evident on mucosal surfaces and thin, nonpigmented skin. When secondary hemostasis is affected, bleeding into body cavities, bruising, ecchymoses, and hematoma formation without recognized trauma is more common. The clinical signs depend on the body cavity affected (ie, cardiac tamponade with pericardial effusion or tachypnea with hemothorax) and the amount of blood that has been lost (ie, hemorrhagic/hypovolemic shock).

In horses, hereditary conditions that result in hypocoagulation are rare. Reported conditions include Glanzmann thrombasthenia,[18,19] platelet fibrinogen binding deficiency,[20,21] prekallikrein deficiency,[22,23] and deficiencies in factors VIII, IX, and X.[24–27]

Excessive thrombosis

When thrombosis occurs, physical examination findings may be obvious or limited. Signs may be related to the thrombus itself or to the effects of the thrombus on blood flow. Arterial thrombi stop blood flow to the region the artery supplies. If collateral circulation is insufficient, the region becomes cold and organ function is compromised. Venous thrombi increase venous backpressure. If collateral circulation or lymphatic drainage is insufficient, it results in edema formation and potential organ dysfunction. The ability to identify signs such as changes in temperature, edema, and organ function depends on the location of the vessel affected. If the thrombosis occurs in a superficial vessel, heat, pain, and swelling at the site of the thrombus can occur depending on how much underlying local inflammation (infectious or noninfectious) is present.

DIC

DIC has a wide range of clinical signs, and diagnosis is based on the presence of a predisposing disease process and clinical pathology findings. Signs of coagulopathy may be nonexistent (subclinical/nonovert DIC) or consistent with systemic excessive thrombosis (multiorgan dysfunction) or excessive bleeding as consumption occurs.

Underlying Disease

Given the frequency of concurrent/underlying diseases associated with coagulopathies, many clinical findings in horses with coagulopathies are related to the underlying disease. In horses, coagulopathy has been most frequently evaluated and documented associated with gastrointestinal disease and neonatal sepsis.[14–17,28–43] Changes in coagulation and fibrinolysis have been associated with morbidity[32,37,42,43] and mortality[14,15,28–30,32,37–41] in horses presenting with gastrointestinal disease. An association between changes in coagulation and fibrinolysis and death has also been reported in septic foals.[33,35]

Studies and reports on thrombosis in horses illustrate an association with inflammatory disease processes. Endotoxemia, hypoproteinemia, large intestinal disease, treatment with antidiarrheal or antiulcerative medications, and salmonellosis have been identified as risk factors for catheter-related jugular vein thrombosis.[44] Jugular thrombophlebitis is more likely to occur in horses with surgically treated colic if they develop fever or diarrhea.[45] Case reports and series describing aortoiliac and limb artery thrombosis have included foals with colitis and septicemia and an adult horse with colitis.[46–48] Massive pulmonary thromboembolism has been reported in horses with strangulating gastrointestinal disease, colitis, retained placenta, myonecrosis, and pneumonia and in a septic foal.[34,49–51]

DIAGNOSTICS
Clinical Pathology

There are large numbers of laboratory tests for coagulation and fibrinolysis, from individual factors to whole-blood viscoelastic testing, which have been evaluated in horses. Evaluation of most horses with coagulopathy or suspected coagulopathy begins with a coagulation panel. Although individual laboratories may have more or less tests in their coagulation panel, the author considers platelet count, PT, aPTT, AT level, fibrinogen level, and FDPs or D-dimers to be a good place to start. Depending on the clinical signs and results of the coagulation panel, additional tests can be selected.

There are significant limitations to the clinical utility of many of these tests. Almost all tests evaluate only portions, or even single elements, of the hemostatic process. None of the tests can take into account the critical role of the endothelium in hemostasis. This deficiency makes it difficult to interpret the effect of identified abnormalities in vivo. Clinical use is also limited by restrictions in availability. Although some of the tests can be performed if samples are sent to specific laboratories, others require rapid processing and can only be performed at hospitals that have the testing equipment. In addition, many tests have wide normal ranges that overlap significantly with results found in diseased horses.

Table 1 summarizes selected tests that have been evaluated in horses. A brief description, interpretation, and limitations of the test are given.

Other Tests

Buccal mucosal bleeding time and template bleeding time (TBT) are additional tests that are performed to diagnose thrombocytopenia and thrombocytopathia. These tests involve creating wounds of specific dimension and depth on either the oral mucosa or skin and then measuring the time until bleeding stops. TBT has been evaluated in horses on the medial side of the antebrachium. However, the study revealed poor reproducibility of the test in horses.[52]

Imaging studies may be useful in locating sites of hemorrhage or thrombosis. In cases of excessive bleeding involving body cavities, ultrasonography may help provide a diagnosis and direct sample collection. In cases of thrombosis,

Table 1
Selected tests of coagulation and fibrinolysis in horses

Test	Description	Interpretation	Limitations
Platelet count	Automated, manual (hemocytometer), or estimated	• Decreased production • Increased destruction • Increased consumption	EDTA can result in pseudothrombocytopenia Pseudothrombocytopenia should be suspected when clumping is evident on cytologic examination Pseudothrombocytopenia can be ruled out by repeating the platelet count on citrated blood
PT	Tests extrinsic and common pathway by adding thromboplastin (TF), Ca^{2+}, and phospholipid to fresh or frozen plasma	• 120% upper end of normal • Decreased amount or activity of FVII, X, V, II, or I • Implied hypercoagulability and consumption	Low PT cannot be interpreted
aPTT	Tests intrinsic and common pathway by adding FXII activator (ellagic acid, kaolin, silica, or celite), Ca^{2+}, and phospholipid to fresh or frozen plasma	• 120% upper end of normal • Decreased amount or activity of prekallikrein, HMWK, FXII, XI, IX, VIII, X, V, II, or I • Implied hypercoagulability and consumption	Low aPTT cannot be interpreted
AT	Measures percentage activity by adding excess heparin and FXa	• Risk for increased clotting • Gastrointestinal or renal loss • Consumption with hypercoagulability	
Fibrinogen	Quantitative (von Clauss and modified PT) and semiquantitative (heat denaturation) methods available	• Inflammation • Consumption with hypercoagulability	Inflammatory nature of underlying disease in most horses with DIC makes hypofibrinogenemia an uncommon finding
FDP	Measure products of degradation of fibrin and fibrinogen	• Increased fibrinolysis implies hypercoagulation/increased clot formation • Hyperfibrinogenemia	Not specific for degradation of cross-linked fibrin (ie, fibrin that was part of a clot) Limited availability of assay Largely replaced by D-dimers

Test	Description	Interpretation	Availability/Notes
D-dimers	Measure product of degradation of cross-linked fibrin (fibrin that was part of a clot)	• Increased fibrinolysis implies hypercoagulation/increased clot formation	Sensitive → increased in pathologic and nonpathologic (ie, surgery) causes of clotting
Activated clotting time	Whole blood collected into tube with diatomaceous earth (parts of intrinsic and common pathways) Time to clot at body temperature Rapid, stall-side test	• Decrease amount or activity of FIX, VIII, II, or I	Not as sensitive as aPTT
Individual clotting factors	Modifications of PT or aPTT or chromogenic detection of activated factor Available for most factors	• Decrease amount or activity of individual factors	Limited availability Rare indications
Thrombin-antithrombin complex	Thrombin bound to antithrombin Cleared rapidly	• Hypercoagulability	Not available for clinical use
PC	Total concentration and functional activity assays available	• Risk for increased clotting • Consumption with hypercoagulability	Not available for clinical use
vWF	Measures percentage activity	• Decreased activity will impair primary hemostasis	Limited availability
Platelet function analyzer-100	Measures time for platelet plug to stop flow of blood through a small hole in a collagen or epinephrine and ADP-impregnated membrane	• Thrombocytopenia • Thrombocytopathia	Limited availability Must be performed within ~4 h of collection
Platelet aggregometry	Stimulated (eg, ADP, collagen, thrombin) aggregation of platelet-rich plasma Rate and degree of aggregation measured	• Thrombocytopathia	Limited availability Must be performed within ~4 h of collection
Viscoelastic coagulation testing (thrombelastography, thrombelastometry, and Sonoclot)	Measure changes in strength of a clot during formation and fibrinolysis over time Uses citrated whole blood → evaluates cellular and enzymatic components of coagulation Can be performed with or without an activator (eg, TF, kaolin, glass beads)	• Hypercoagulability or hypocoagulability associated with changes in primary or secondary hemostasis • Hyperfibrinolysis or hypofibrinolysis	Limited availability Must be performed approximately 30 min after collection

Abbreviations: EDTA, ethylenediaminetetraacetic acid; HMWK, high molecular weight kininogen.

ultrasonography, venography or arteriography, nuclear scintigraphy, thermography, computed tomography, and magnetic resonance imaging may be helpful in locating and characterizing thrombosis and areas of ischemia.

Decision Algorithms

When presented with a horse that has excessive bleeding, a simple algorithm is used to determine the cause of the bleeding or direct further testing based on the results of a coagulation panel (platelet count, PT, aPTT, AT, fibrinogen, and FDPs or D-dimers).

- Is the platelet count normal?
  - Yes
    - Are the PT, aPTT, AT, fibrinogen, and FDPs/D-dimers normal?
      - Yes
        - Suggestive of thrombocytopathia
        - Consider platelet function analyzer-100 or platelet aggregation
        - Is the horse on any medications that could interfere with platelet function (eg, nonsteroidal antiinflammatory drugs, aspirin, clopidogrel, hydroxyethyl starches)?
      - No
        - Less than or equal to 2 abnormal values
          - Abnormal PT or aPTT alone
            - Suggestive of individual clotting factor deficiency or dysfunction
            - Consider testing for individual clotting factor deficiencies or dysfunction
            - Is the horse on any drugs or has it been exposed to any toxins that could interfere with secondary hemostasis (eg, heparin, vitamin K antagonists)?
          - Abnormal FDP/D-dimers alone
            - May be result of inflammatory disease or normal activation of coagulation
          - Alternatively, consider subclinical/nonovert DIC
            - Look for appropriate underlying disease
            - Three or more abnormal values
            - Suggestive of DIC
            - Look for appropriate underlying disease
  - No
    - Are the PT, aPTT, AT, fibrinogen, and FDPs/D-dimers normal?
      - Yes
        - Diagnosis of thrombocytopenia
        - Perform diagnostic testing to determine the cause of the thrombocytopenia (eg, immune mediated, drug associated, toxic)
      - No
        - Consumptive coagulopathy
          - Primary thrombocytopenia causing bleeding and consumption of soluble factors (generally platelet count ≤10,000–20,000 cells/µL)
            - Perform diagnostics to determine the cause of the thrombocytopenia
          - Secondary consumptive thrombocytopenia (generally platelet count >20,000 cells/µL) caused by bleeding associated with deficiency or dysfunction of an individual clotting factor or DIC (clinical or subclinical)

- Consider testing for individual clotting factor deficiencies or dysfunction
- Look for appropriate underlying disease for DIC

When presented with a horse that has excessive thrombosis, diagnosis is often difficult if the thrombosis is widespread. If thrombosis is localized, an inciting cause, such as infection or trauma (ie, catheterization), should be suspected. With widespread thrombosis, the following algorithm is used to help categorize the disorder or direct further testing based on the results of a coagulation panel (platelet count, PT, aPTT, AT, fibrinogen, and FDPs or D-dimers).

- Is the coagulation panel normal?
  - Yes
    - Is the cause hypercoagulation, hypofibrinolysis, or decreased anticoagulants?
      - Consider viscoelastic testing for hypercoagulation and hypofibrinolysis
      - Consider testing for decreased PC
  - No
    - Abnormal AT alone
      - Look for gastrointestinal or renal AT loss
    - Multiple abnormal parameters
      - Suggestive of DIC
      - Implies hypercoagulability has resulted in consumption of platelets and coagulation and anticoagulation factors and production of fibrinolytic products
      - Consider viscoelastic testing for hypercoagulation and hypofibrinolysis
      - Look for appropriate underlying cause

TREATMENT OPTIONS

When determining the course of treatment of a horse with a coagulopathy, it is important to remember that primary coagulopathies are rare in horses. For this reason, therapy should always include treatment of any underlying disease, stopping/removing any predisposing treatments (ie, anticoagulants, hydroxyethylstarches,[53] jugular catheters), and identifying and treating any toxins (ie, rodenticides). In addition, many horses have coagulopathies that are subclinical/nonovert and, therefore, have no clinical signs (excessive bleeding or thrombosis). Because the process of hemostasis is complicated and it is difficult to predict the in vivo implications of coagulation testing, treatment with drugs that affect coagulation and fibrinolysis should be done cautiously.

For Excessive Bleeding

Treatment of horses with excessive bleeding depends on the location and extent of bleeding. In all cases, systemic administration of procoagulants and antifibrinolytics may be useful. If the location of the bleeding is surgically accessible and the patient can be stabilized enough to undergo surgery (standing or under general anesthesia), then surgical methods of hemostasis and topical hemostatic agents can be used. **Table 2** summarizes selected treatments for excessive bleeding.

For Excessive Thrombosis

Treatment of horses with excessive thrombosis depends on the location and extent of bleeding. If a single-vessel thrombosis is suspected and surgically accessible (with or without interventional radiology), thrombectomy can be considered to return normal

Table 2
Selected treatments for excessive bleeding

Treatment	Mechanism of Action	Dose	Other
Oxidized regenerated cellulose	Swells as soaked with blood → provides pressure over area of bleeding Surface activates coagulation Low pH is caustic	Topical → N/A	Low pH makes antibacterial[54] Low pH makes inflammatory → remove excess
Purified gelatin sponge	Swells as soaked with blood → provides pressure over area of bleeding	Topical → N/A	Avoid in contaminated wounds Can soak in thrombin[55]
Microfibrillar collagen agents (flour, sheet, sponge)	Bind to bleeding surface Collagen activates platelets	Topical → N/A	Can interfere with wound healing and bacterial clearance → remove[55] Less effective with thrombocytopenia[56]
Polysaccharide hemostatic agents (spheres, impregnated dressing)	Absorb blood and concentrate platelets and coagulation factors	Topical → N/A	May not be as effective for severe bleeding as other topicals
Thrombin products (variety of preparations)	Converts fibrinogen to fibrin Activates platelets	Topical → N/A	Antibody formation has been reported in humans
Fibrin-based sealants (fibrinogen and thrombin)	Adhere to tissue and form a fibrin clot	Topical → N/A	Can be used in patients with primary and secondary hemostasis deficiencies

Therapy	Mechanism	Dose	Comments
Antifibrinolytics (ε-aminocaproic acid [EACA], tranexamic acid [TEA])	Inhibit plasminogen activator activity. Stimulate release of α2-antiplasmin → direct inhibition plasmin[57]	EACA • 20–40 mg/kg in 1 L 0.9% NaCl IV q6h[58] • 3.5 mg/kg/min for 15 min, then 0.25 mg/kg/min CRI[59] • Topical application[60] TEA • 5–25 mg/kg IV, IM, SC q12h[58]	The therapeutic plasma levels for EACA and TEA seem lower than for humans[61]. Studies on TEA limited, dose empirically derived
Yunnan Bia Yao	Largely unknown. Proposed mechanism involves saponins activating platelets[62,63]	4 g PO q6h. Topical application	Studies in horses limited
Estrogen	Increases clotting factors VII, X, and fibrinogen. Increased platelet activity[64]	0.05 mg/kg[65]	No information available in horses
Whole blood or fresh plasma	Provides platelet and clotting factors	Unknown/variable	Only therapy that contains platelets. Also contains anticoagulants, fibrinolytic proteins, cytokines
Fresh frozen plasma	Provides clotting factors	Unknown/variable	Also contains anticoagulants, fibrinolytic proteins, cytokines
Vitamin K	Required for synthesis of FII, VII, IX, X (and proteins C and S)	0.5–2.5 mg/kg IV, IM, SC[58]	Indicated if deficiency or antagonist toxicity
Naloxone	Antagonizes endogenous opioid induced vasodilation	0.2 mg/kg IV[66]	Adjunctive therapy for hemorrhagic shock

Abbreviations: CRI, constant rate infusion; IM, intramuscularly; IV, intravenously; N/A, not applicable; PO, by mouth; q6h, every 6 hours; SC, subcutaneously.

Table 3
Selected treatments for excessive thrombosis

Treatment	Mechanism of Action	Dose	Other
Low-molecular-weight heparin	Binds to AT and potentiates inhibition of activated clotting factors	Dalteparin • Adult—50 IU/kg SC SID[68]–BID[69] • Foals—100 IU/kg SC SID[70] Enoxaparin • Adult—40 IU/kg SC SID[68]	Specifically binds to FXa Less side effects and more predictable dose response[71] Difficult to monitor with aPTT; requires measurement of anti-Xa activity or possibly viscoelastic coagulation testing[72] Decreased jugular vein thrombosis compared with unfractionated heparin[73]
Unfractionated heparin	Binds to AT and potentiates inhibition of activated clotting factors	40–60 IU IV, SC q8-12h	Less-specific inhibition of FXa Degree and duration of effect unpredictable[71] Red blood cell agglutination and decreased platelet count possible[74]
Clopidogrel	Platelet ADP receptor (P2Y$_{12}$) inhibitor	2 mg/kg PO SID	At 2 mg/kg PO decreased platelet aggregation was delayed but long lasting,[75] suggesting a loading dose may be required for more rapid therapy
Aspirin	Inhibits cyclooxygenase→in platelets prevents TxA$_2$ production	10–100 mg/kg PO SID-EOD 20 mg/kg per rectum q12 h	As low as 5 mg/kg PO inhibits TxA$_2$ but not platelet aggregation[75] 11 mg/kg PO decreased platelet aggregation[76]

Abbreviations: BID, twice a day; EOD, every other day; IV, intravenously; PO, by mouth; q8-12h, every 8 to 12 hours; q12h, every 12 hours; SC, subcutaneously; SID, once a day.

blood flow. This technique has been used with some success in horses with aortoiliac thrombosis.[67] Although not reported in horses, local administration of a fibrinolytic agent such as tPA could also be considered. Systemic anticoagulants can be used in cases of local or widespread thrombotic disease. **Table 3** summarizes selected treatments for excessive thrombosis.

REFERENCES

1. Frenette PS, Johnson RC, Hynes RO, et al. Platelets roll on stimulated endothelium in vivo: an interaction mediated by endothelial P-selectin. Proc Natl Acad Sci U S A 1995;92(16):7450–4.
2. Thomas S. Platelet membrane glycoproteins in haemostasis. Clin Lab 2002; 48(5–6):247–62.
3. McMichael M. Primary hemostasis. J Vet Emerg Crit Care (San Antonio) 2005;15: 1–8.
4. Ashby B, Colman R, Daniel J, et al. Platelet stimulatory and inhibitory receptors. In: Colman R, Hirsh J, Marder VJ, et al, editors. Hemostasis and thrombosis basic principles and clinical practice. 2001. p. 505–20.
5. Ruggeri ZM. Von Willebrand factor, platelets and endothelial cell interactions. J Thromb Haemost 2003;1(7):1335–42.
6. Smith SA. The cell-based model of coagulation. J Vet Emerg Crit Care (San Antonio) 2009;19(1):3–10.
7. Roemisch J, Gray E, Hoffmann JN, et al. Antithrombin: a new look at the actions of a serine protease inhibitor. Blood Coagul Fibrinolysis 2002;13(8):657–70.
8. Esmon CT. Protein C, protein S, and thrombomodulin. In: Colman R, Hirsh J, Marder VJ, et al, editors. Hemostasis and thrombosis: basic principles and clinical practice. 4th edition; 2001. p. 335–53.
9. Broze GJ Jr. Tissue factor pathway inhibitor and the revised theory of coagulation. Annu Rev Med 1995;46:103–12.
10. Levy JH, Dutton RP, Hemphill JC 3rd, et al. Multidisciplinary approach to the challenge of hemostasis. Anesth Analg 2010;110(2):354–64.
11. Whitta RK, Cox DJ, Mallett SV. Thrombelastography reveals two causes of haemorrhage in HELLP syndrome. Br J Anaesth 1995;74(4):464–8.
12. Dallap Schaer BL, Epstein K. Coagulopathy of the critically ill equine patient. J Vet Emerg Crit Care (San Antonio) 2009;19(1):53–65.
13. Taylor FB Jr, Toh CH, Hoots WK, et al. Towards definition, clinical and laboratory criteria, and a scoring system for disseminated intravascular coagulation. Thromb Haemost 2001;86(5):1327–30.
14. Dolente BA, Wilkins PA, Boston RC. Clinicopathologic evidence of disseminated intravascular coagulation in horses with acute colitis. J Am Vet Med Assoc 2002; 220(7):1034–8.
15. Dallap BL, Dolente B, Boston R. Coagulation profiles in 27 horses with large colon volvulus. J Vet Emerg Crit Care (San Antonio) 2003;13(4):215–25.
16. Cotovio M, Monreal L, Navarro M, et al. Detection of fibrin deposits in tissues from horses with severe gastrointestinal disorders. J Vet Intern Med 2007; 21(2):308–13.
17. Cotovio M, Monreal L, Armengou L, et al. Fibrin deposits and organ failure in newborn foals with severe septicemia. J Vet Intern Med 2008;22(6): 1403–10.
18. Macieira S, Rivard GE, Champagne J, et al. Glanzmann thrombasthenia in an Oldenbourg filly. Vet Clin Pathol 2007;36(2):204–8.

19. Christopherson PW, van Santen VL, Livesey L, et al. A 10-base-pair deletion in the gene encoding platelet glycoprotein IIb associated with Glanzmann thrombasthenia in a horse. J Vet Intern Med 2007;21(1):196–8.
20. Norris JW, Pratt SM, Auh JH, et al. Investigation of a novel, heritable bleeding diathesis of thoroughbred horses and development of a screening assay. J Vet Intern Med 2006;20(6):1450–6.
21. Norris JW, Pratt SM, Hunter JF, et al. Prevalence of reduced fibrinogen binding to platelets in a population of Thoroughbreds. Am J Vet Res 2007;68(7):716–21.
22. Goer RJ, Jakson ML, Lewis KD, et al. Prekallikrein deficiency in a family of Belgian horses. J Am Vet Med Assoc 1990;197:741.
23. Turrentine MA, Sculley PW, Green EM, et al. Prekallikrein deficiency in a family of miniature horses. Am J Vet Res 1986;47(11):2464–7.
24. Hinton M, Jones DR, Lewis IM, et al. A clotting defect in an Arab colt foal. Equine Vet J 1977;9(1):1–3.
25. Littlewood JD, Bevan SA, Corke MJ. Haemophilia A (classic haemophilia, factor VIII deficiency) in a Thoroughbred colt foal. Equine Vet J 1991;23(1):70–2.
26. Henninger RW. Hemophilia A in two related quarter horse colts. J Am Vet Med Assoc 1988;193(1):91–4.
27. Mills JN, Bolton JR. Haemophilia A in a 3-year-old thoroughbred horse. Aust Vet J 1983;60(2):63–4.
28. Topper MJ, Prasse KW. Use of enzyme-linked immunosorbent assay to measure thrombin-antithrombin III complexes in horses with colic. Am J Vet Res 1996;57(4):456–62.
29. Darien BJ, Potempa J, Moore JN, et al. Antithrombin III activity in horses with colic: an analysis of 46 cases. Equine Vet J 1991;23(3):211–4.
30. Johnstone IB, Crane S. Haemostatic abnormalities in horses with colic–their prognostic value. Equine Vet J 1986;18(4):271–4.
31. Dallap BL, Dolente B, Boston R. Hemostatic and fibrinolytic indices in neonatal foals with presumed septicemia. J Vet Emerg Crit Care (San Antonio) 2003;13(4):215–25.
32. Epstein KL, Brainard BM, Giguere S, et al. Serial viscoelastic and traditional coagulation testing in horses with gastrointestinal disease. J Vet Emerg Crit Care (San Antonio) 2013;23(5):504–16.
33. Dallap Schaer BL, Bentz AI, Boston RC, et al. Comparison of viscoelastic coagulation analysis and standard coagulation profiles in critically ill neonatal foals to outcome. J Vet Emerg Crit Care (San Antonio) 2009;19(1):88–95.
34. Barton MH, Morris DD, Norton N, et al. Hemostatic and fibrinolytic indices in neonatal foals with presumed septicemia. J Vet Intern Med 1998;12(1):26–35.
35. Armengou L, Monreal L, Tarancon I, et al. Plasma D-dimer concentration in sick newborn foals. J Vet Intern Med 2008;22(2):411–7.
36. Mendez-Angulo JL, Mudge M, Zaldivar-Lopez S, et al. Thromboelastography in healthy, sick non-septic and septic neonatal foals. Aust Vet J 2011;89(12):500–5.
37. Epstein KL, Brainard BM, Gomez-Ibanez SE, et al. Thrombelastography in horses with acute gastrointestinal disease. J Vet Intern Med 2011;25(2):307–14.
38. Collatos C, Barton MH, Moore JN. Fibrinolytic activity in plasma from horses with gastrointestinal diseases: changes associated with diagnosis, surgery, and outcome. J Vet Intern Med 1995;9(1):18–23.
39. Collatos C, Barton MH, Prasse KW, et al. Intravascular and peritoneal coagulation and fibrinolysis in horses with acute gastrointestinal tract diseases. J Am Vet Med Assoc 1995;207(4):465–70.

40. Henry MM, Moore JN. Whole blood re-calcification time in equine colic. Equine Vet J 1991;23(4):303–8.

41. Sandholm M, Vidovic A, Puotunen-Reinert A, et al. D-dimer improves the prognostic value of combined clinical and laboratory data in equine gastrointestinal colic. Acta Vet Scand 1995;36(2):255–72.

42. Welles EG, Prasse KW, Moore JN. Use of newly developed assays for protein C and plasminogen in horses with signs of colic. Am J Vet Res 1991;52(2): 345–51.

43. Prasse KW, Topper MJ, Moore JN, et al. Analysis of hemostasis in horses with colic. J Am Vet Med Assoc 1993;203(5):685–93.

44. Dolente BA, Beech J, Lindborg S, et al. Evaluation of risk factors for development of catheter-associated jugular thrombophlebitis in horses: 50 cases (1993-1998). J Am Vet Med Assoc 2005;227(7):1134–41.

45. Lankveld DP, Ensink JM, van Dijk P, et al. Factors influencing the occurrence of thrombophlebitis after post-surgical long-term intravenous catheterization of colic horses: a study of 38 cases. J Vet Med A Physiol Pathol Clin Med 2001; 48(9):545–52.

46. Brainceau P, Divers TJ. Acute thrombosis of limb arteries in horses with sepsis: five cases (1988-1998). Equine Vet J 2001;33:105–9.

47. Breshears MA, Holbrook TC, Haak CE, et al. Pulmonary aspergillosis and ischemic distal limb necrosis associated with enteric salmonellosis in a foal. Vet Pathol 2007;44(2):215–7.

48. Moore LA, Johnson PJ, Bailey KL. Aorto-iliac thrombosis in a foal. Vet Rec 1998; 142(17):459–62.

49. Norman TE, Chaffin MK, Perris EE, et al. Massive pulmonary thromboembolism in six horses. Equine Vet J 2008;40(5):514–7.

50. Carr EA, Carlson GP, Wilson WD, et al. Acute hemorrhagic pulmonary infarction and necrotizing pneumonia in horses: 21 cases (1967-1993). J Am Vet Med Assoc 1997;210(12):1774–8.

51. Ryu SH, Kim JG, Bak UB, et al. A hematogenic pleuropneumonia caused by postoperative septic thrombophlebitis in a Thoroughbred gelding. J Vet Sci 2004;5(1):75–7.

52. Segura D, Monreal L. Poor reproducibility of template bleeding time in horses. J Vet Intern Med 2008;22(1):238–41.

53. Blong AE, Epstein KL, Brainard BM. In vitro effects of three formulations of hydroxyethyl starch solutions on coagulation and platelet function in horses. Am J Vet Res 2013;74(5):712–20.

54. Spangler D, Rothenburger S, Nguyen K, et al. In vitro antimicrobial activity of oxidized regenerated cellulose against antibiotic-resistant microorganisms. Surg Infect (Larchmt) 2003;4(3):255–62.

55. Schonauer C, Tessitore E, Barbagallo G, et al. The use of local agents: bone wax, gelatin, collagen, oxidized cellulose. Eur Spine J 2004;13(Suppl 1):S89–96.

56. Boucher BA, Traub O. Achieving hemostasis in the surgical field. Pharmacotherapy 2009;29(7 Pt 2):2S–7S.

57. Ray MJ, Hales M, Marsh N. Epsilon-aminocaproic acid promotes the release of alpha2-antiplasmin during and after cardiopulmonary bypass. Blood Coagul Fibrinolysis 2001;12(2):129–35.

58. Appendix. In: Corley K, Stephen J, editors. The equine hospital manual. Oxford: Blackwell Publishing; 2008.

59. Ross J, Dallap BL, Dolente BA, et al. Pharmacokinetics and pharmacodynamics of epsilon-aminocaproic acid in horses. Am J Vet Res 2007;68(9):1016–21.

60. Gurian DB, Meneghini A, de Abreu LC, et al. A randomized trial of the topical effect of antifibrinolytic epsilon aminocaproic acid on coronary artery bypass surgery without cardiopulmonary bypass. Clin Appl Thromb Hemost 2013. [Epub ahead of print].

61. Fletcher DJ, Brainard BM, Epstein K, et al. Therapeutic plasma concentrations of epsilon aminocaproic acid and tranexamic acid in horses. J Vet Intern Med 2013;27:1589–95.

62. Liu XX, Wang L, Chen XQ, et al. Simultaneous quantification of both triterpenoid and steroidal saponins in various Yunnan Baiyao preparations using HPLC-UV and HPLC-MS. J Sep Sci 2008;31(22):3834–46.

63. Chew EC. Effects of Yunnan Bai Yao on blood platelets: an ultrastructural study. Comp Med East West 1977;5(2):169–75.

64. Norris LA, Bonnar J. Haemostatic changes and the oral contraceptive pill. Baillieres Clin Obstet Gynaecol 1997;11(3):545–64.

65. Steiner JV, Hillman RB, Orsini JA, et al. Reproductive system. In: Orsini JA, Divers TJ, editors. Equine emergencies: treatment and procedures. 3rd edition. Saunders: St Louis; 2008. p. 411–34.

66. Weld JM, Kamerling SG, Combie JD, et al. The effects of naloxone on endotoxic and hemorrhagic shock in horses. Res Commun Chem Pathol Pharmacol 1984; 44(2):227–38.

67. Rijkenhuizen AB, Sinclair D, Jahn W. Surgical thrombectomy in horses with aortoiliac thrombosis: 17 cases. Equine Vet J 2009;41(8):754–8.

68. Schwarzwald CC, Feige K, Wunderli-Allenspach H, et al. Comparison of pharmacokinetic variables for two low-molecular-weight heparins after subcutaneous administration of a single dose to horses. Am J Vet Res 2002;63(6):868–73.

69. Whelchel DD, Tennent-Brown BS, Giguere S, et al. Pharmacodynamics of multidose low molecular weight heparin in healthy horses. Vet Surg 2013;42(4): 448–54.

70. Armengou L, Monreal L, Delgado MA, et al. Low-molecular-weight heparin dosage in newborn foals. J Vet Intern Med 2010;24(5):1190–5.

71. Boneu B. Low molecular weight heparin therapy: is monitoring needed? Thromb Haemost 1994;72(3):330–4.

72. Tennent-Brown BS, Epstein KL, Whelchel DD, et al. Use of viscoelastic coagulation testing to monitor low molecular weight heparin administration to healthy horses. J Vet Emerg Crit Care (San Antonio) 2013;23(3):291–9.

73. Feige K, Schwarzwald CC, Bombeli T. Comparison of unfractioned and low molecular weight heparin for prophylaxis of coagulopathies in 52 horses with colic: a randomised double-blind clinical trial. Equine Vet J 2003;35(5):506–13.

74. Monreal L, Villatoro AJ, Monreal M, et al. Comparison of the effects of low-molecular-weight and unfractioned heparin in horses. Am J Vet Res 1995; 56(10):1281–5.

75. Brainard BM, Epstein KL, LoBato D, et al. Effects of clopidogrel and aspirin on platelet aggregation, thromboxane production, and serotonin secretion in horses. J Vet Intern Med 2011;25(1):116–22.

76. Cambridge H, Lees P, Hooke RE, et al. Antithrombotic actions of aspirin in the horse. Equine Vet J 1991;23(2):123–7.

Trauma and Wound Management

Gunshot Wounds in Horses

Amelia S. Munsterman, DVM, MS*, R. Reid Hanson, DVM

KEYWORDS

- Equine • Penetrating trauma • Gunshot • Bullet wounds

KEY POINTS

- Gunshot injury in horses is classified as a penetrating type of trauma.
- The severity of gunshot wounds depends on the kinetic energy of the bullet on impact, the type of bullet, and the characteristics of the tissue it passes through.
- Elastic and cohesive tissues, including muscle, lung, blood vessels, and nerves, may recover after a gunshot wound, whereas less cohesive or elastic organs, such as liver, brain, heart, and bone, are less likely to survive.
- The bullet is not sterilized by the heat of the impact, so gunshot wounds should be treated as contaminated.

INTRODUCTION

Although gunshot injuries in horses are uncommon, they can result in a diverse array of traumatic injuries because of the indiscriminate nature of where the bullets strike. Bullet wounds are described as a focal, penetrating trauma, and may affect skin and superficial structures, musculoskeletal tissues, as well as internal organs and neurovascular structures. The physical appearance of the entry wound is often oval to circular, with clean margins (**Fig. 1**). There may be a hyperemic ring surrounding the entrance, caused by local inflammation or from direct damage by carbon monoxide released from the gun barrel if the animal was shot at close range. High-velocity impacts are similar to small explosions, causing a vacuum to form in the tissues as the bullet passes through. In these cases, foreign material may be sucked into the exit wound. For close-range shotgun injuries, total tissue destruction is the norm.[1,2]

No funding applicable.
The authors have nothing to disclose.
Department of Clinical Sciences, J.T. Vaughan Large Animal Teaching Hospital, Auburn University College of Veterinary Medicine, 1500 Wire Road, Auburn, AL 36849, USA
* Corresponding author.
E-mail address: munstas@auburn.edu

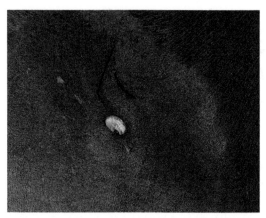

Fig. 1. A 12-year old quarter horse hit by a ricochet from a rifle shot in the ventral abdomen. The entry wound is circumscribed and distinct. No exit wound was found, consistent with a low-energy impact. The ventral colon was perforated in 2 sites causing a peritonitis (gunshot wound score from **Table 2**: LE-S, V-3, W-2, F-0, C-3).

CLASSIFICATION OF WOUNDING POTENTIAL

In the past, bullet wounds were categorized by the firearm that discharged the bullet, but this vague classification has been redefined by a better understanding of ballistics, which is the study of the movement of projectiles, as well as the types of weapons commonly available to civilian populations. The wounding potential of a bullet is now described in relation to 3 factors that affect the amount of damaging energy transferred to the tissues. These factors are the energy of the missile on impact, the design of the bullet, and the characteristics of the tissues involved. The practitioner should become familiar with these principles to understand the nature of the injury and to provide appropriate care for the wound.

IMPACT ENERGY

Firearms are traditionally grouped into 3 major types based on the speed of the projectile at the time it leaves the barrel, called the muzzle velocity. This velocity is the sum of the forward and rotational energies that propel the projectile forward.[3] Low-velocity firearms, including handguns, are those that fire projectiles at a muzzle velocity of less than 350 m/s (1148 feet/s). Medium-velocity projectiles are fired at 350–600 m/s (1148–1968 feet/s), and include weapons such as shotguns and magnum handguns, whereas high-velocity weapons, such as military-grade weapons and hunting rifles, fire at greater than 600 m/s (>1968 feet/s) (**Table 1**). A longer barrel imparts a higher velocity to the bullet, by increasing acceleration by expansion of gases; conversely a shorter barrel imparts a lower speed to the projectile.[4] All of these types of weapons have been reported to cause equine gunshot wounds.[5,6]

Although it is tempting to describe the trauma caused by a bullet based on the initial muzzle velocity alone, this is the maximum speed the bullet reaches during flight. Multiple factors, including the bullet's shape and the distance the bullet travels, can slow the speed and reduce the energy of the projectile on impact. The muzzle velocity is significantly reduced at distances greater than 45 m with low-velocity firearms, whereas projectiles from high-velocity firearms are slowed significantly at distances greater than 90 m.[3] Shotguns are particularly susceptible to the effects of distance,

Table 1
Classification of firearms based on muzzle velocity

Firearm Classification	Muzzle Velocity	Examples of Weapon
Low-velocity firearms	<350 m/s	.22 Long Rifle .38 Special revolver Colt .45 revolver
Medium-velocity firearms	350–600 m/s	.375 Sig Sauer pistol .357 Magnum revolver .44 Magnum revolver .50 caliber revolver
High-velocity firearms	>600 m/s	.223 Remington rifle .30–30 Winchester rifle .30–06 Springfield rifle

because of the poor aerodynamics of the individual pellets released from the cartridge.[7] At close range (<5 m), these projectiles can act as 1 unit and move at speeds similar to those produced by a high-velocity firearm (**Fig. 2**). At distances greater than 5 m, the scatter and loss of kinetic energy significantly reduce tissue penetration, often resulting in only superficial damage to skin and fascia.

The bullet speed can also be affected by objects it encounters or impacts before tissue wounding. This interference can alter the angle of the bullet between its longitudinal axis and its path of flight, termed the yaw of the bullet.[8,9] The yaw is normally affected by the bullet's center of mass as well as the spin on the bullet. The bullet

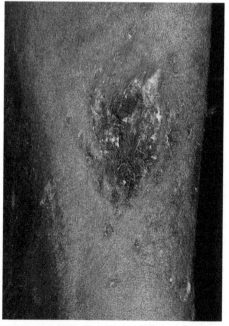

Fig. 2. Close-range (<5 m) gunshot wound to a cadaveric distal tibia using a Winchester 12-gauge shotgun (30-g [1 1/16 oz] waterfowl steel shot). The pellets acted in unison, with little scatter noted in the skin perforations. The distal tibia showed a comminuted fracture (gunshot wound score: HE-C, V-2, W-2, EF-2, C-2).

ideally maintains a yaw of 1 to 5° from its rotational axis, because of the spin imparted by the rifling inside the barrel. The closer the bullet remains to parallel, the less energy is lost during its flight and the longer it can travel. Impact with objects before hitting the target can deform the bullet, changing its angle and reducing its speed, which can decrease the impact energy further.

BULLET DESIGN

Other factors that affect the wounding potential of the bullet include its shape and center of mass, which determine its yaw, and the caliber of the bullet, which is the diameter of the projectile. The caliber of the bullet is directly related to the damage potential, and inversely related to the velocity at which it travels, in that the larger the projectile, the slower a given muzzle energy causes it to move.[3] One caveat to this is the shotgun. With this type of weapon, the total mass of the pellets can increase the kinetic energy, depending on the distance they have to travel; the choke (constriction) in the barrel, which limits spread of the pellets; the gauge of the shotgun; and the size of the pellets.

Regarding the shape of the bullet, there are 3 general classes of projectile: those that are unjacketed or partially jacketed, which are meant to fragment or deform; jacketed projectiles, meant to remain intact; and pellets encased in a shotgun cartridge.[1,10] Jacketed bullets consist of a soft lead or steel core, surrounded by a casing of copper, zinc, or cupronickel alloy. The purpose of the jacket is to prevent fragmentation of the bullet within the barrel at high muzzle velocities. The jacket reduces loss of speed, resulting in full penetration through the target, and reducing deformation or mushrooming. The jacket also decreases yaw through the first portion of the tissue encountered, making the damage path similar between high-velocity and low-velocity bullets by preventing secondary tissue damage caused by tumbling of the projectile. In thicker tissue, yaw may still occur, causing fragmentation and injury to adjacent tissues.

A soft-point or hollow-point bullet is designed to deform or fragment at the top of the bullet on entry.[1] This mushrooming causes an increase in the bullet's surface area or caliber, and increases crushing injury and wounding potential. To do this, the jacket is either missing or only a partial covering to allow exposure of the softer metal within. Some bullets may have only a thin layer of electroplating over the soft core; these are still considered unjacketed. At high speeds, they can be more damaging than jacketed bullets, enlarging the wound path up to 4 times the original diameter of the bullet after deformation and fragmentation.[11] However, the depth of penetration is decreased because of loss of energy caused by the deformation, and depends on the kinetic energy at impact.[10,12] This energy depends on both mass and velocity.

It is hard to identify the type of bullet without direct examination, and deformation of the bullet by impact can make this difficult for clinicians not trained in forensic science. Radiographs cannot differentiate the jacket of a bullet from the soft core if the bullet has not fragmented.[13] Soft-point and hollow-point bullets are also hard to positively identify on radiographs. The bullet may not expand for several reasons, including insufficient velocity, excessively thick or stiff metal jackets, manufacturer differences, or plugging of the hollow point by debris. However, if lead has been exposed on the bullet, it may lose flakes along its path. This loss is noted as a spatter or lead snowstorm, and can help clinicians to differentiate between a jacketed bullet versus a nonjacketed bullet that has not deformed (**Fig. 3**).[1,14] If the bullet does fragment, the jacket may be visible separate from the core, often originating from the back half of the bullet where it is crimped to the cartridge case, called the cannelure.[13]

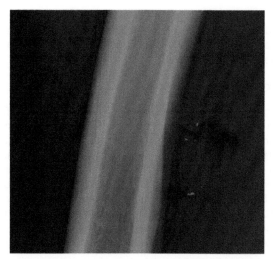

Fig. 3. A lead snowstorm noted in the soft tissues caudal to the radius in a cadaver horse limb hit by two 0.22 caliber bullets from a Ruger 1022 target rifle (.22 Long Rifle, 2.3-g [36-grain] hollow-point bullets). The spatter is caused by exposed lead flaking off the bullet as it traverses the tissues (gunshot wound score: LE-C, V-0, W-3, F-0, C-1).

TISSUES INVOLVED

As mentioned, the type of tissues the bullet encounters affects dissipation of the kinetic energy on impact. Energy dissipation is directly related to the target tissue density, and inversely related to tissue elasticity.[3] Increased density can increase the energy transferred by forcing the bullet to yaw and tumble through the tissue, or by fragmenting the projectiles. Organs with low elasticity include the liver, spleen, great vessels, nerves, and bone, whereas elastic tissues include muscle, skin, and lung. Fluid-filled organs, such as the bladder, heart, and viscera, are classified as elastic but can be secondarily damaged by pressure waves. Once the bullet enters tissues, it can no longer stabilize itself against yaw, especially if unjacketed. If it does not deform on impact, it yaws forward 90°, allowing it to impact more tissues.[4] Whether through yaw, mushrooming of the bullet, or fragmentation, the bullet is slower and the wounding potential depleted as it moves through the target.[12]

The penetrating trauma caused by the bullet induces 2 types of injury.[3,15] First is crush injury, referred to as the permanent cavity formation, which causes direct tissue necrosis. This injury results from the path of the bullet and its fragments, as well as secondary missiles formed from the tissues or objects through which the bullet passes. Crush injuries can be associated with both high-velocity and low-velocity projectiles, because they result directly from the foreign material passing through the tissue. The amount of crush injury depends on the size and shape of the bullet and whether it is designed to fragment or deform on impact.

At higher speeds, large-diameter objects can also cause blunt trauma because of energy displacement into the adjacent tissues. This lateral expansion, termed temporary cavitation, is typically associated with high-caliber handguns or centerfire rifles, in which the primer that ignites the powder is located in the center of the head of the cartridge case. This expansion can be between 10 and 40 times the diameter of the projectile, but is directly related to the type of tissue involved.[4,15] However, if the speed has been significantly reduced by distance traveled or encounters with objects before impact, even a high-velocity bullet will cause only crush injuries in the permanent cavity. Survival of tissues injured by blunt trauma varies depending on the elasticity of the organ involved. Organs that are elastic and cohesive in nature (muscle, lung, blood vessels, and nerves) may recover, whereas less cohesive or elastic organs (liver, brain, heart, bone) are less likely to survive.[10]

BULLET WOUND CLASSIFICATION SYSTEM

In order to determine the severity of equine bullet wounds, a classification system is modeled after the civilian scoring system created by Gugala and Lindsey[3] for human gunshot injuries. In this system, wounds are described based on 5 features to indicate severity, nature of the injury, extent of tissue involved, and clinical significance. Wounds classified as high energy, those with a higher score for vital structures involved, and those with a higher score for contamination may be more likely to require surgical intervention or cause fatality.[16] This system has been modified to describe equine bullet wounds (**Table 2**). Each wound in the figures shown in this article has been graded, and those with scores greater than 7 required surgical intervention. Additional cases are needed to determine the validity of the scoring categories for equine trauma.

ENERGY

Estimating the bullet's energy is important in classification to determine the potential amount of wounding that can be imparted to the tissues involved. In this classification,

Table 2	
Equine gunshot wound scoring system	
E (missile impact energy dissipated in target tissues)	LE-C = 1 HE-C = 2 LE-S = 1 HE-S = 2
V	V = 0, no vital structure injured V = 1, functional damage (nerve injury) V = 2, structural damage (neurovascular) V = 3, injury to viscera, major vessels, CNS
W	W = 1, nonpenetrating W = 2, penetrating W = 3, perforating
F	F = 0, no fracture EF EF = 1, little to no comminution EF = 2, significant comminution IF IF = 1, 1 perforation, minimal soft tissue damage IF = 2, one or more perforations, extensive soft tissue damage IF = 3, open periarticular fracture with articular involvement, dislocation, vascular injury, or nerve injury
C	C = 1, moderately clean wound C = 2, moderately contaminated wound C = 3, gross contamination with visceral contents

Abbreviations: C, contamination; CNS, central nervous system; E, energy; EF, extra-articular fracture; F, fracture; HE-C, high energy confirmed; HE-S, high energy suspected; IF, intra-articular fracture; LE-C, low energy confirmed; LE-S, low energy suspected; V, vital structure; W, wound.

Adapted from Gugala Z, Lindsey RW. Classification of gunshot injuries in civilians. Clin Orthop Relat Res 2003;408:70; with permission.

the energy transferred is related to the type of tissue involved and the distance the bullet traveled through the tissues.[3] Low-energy wounds are classified as those involving nonjacketed bullets, traveling in short wound tracts through low-density, elastic tissues (skin, adipose, or muscle). In these wounds, the trauma is mainly caused by cutting and crushing in the path of the projectile. High-energy wounds involve structures farther from the primary bullet tract, caused by shockwaves and temporary cavitation. High-energy wounds are usually inflicted by firearms at close range (<90 m) or shotguns at distances less than 5 m, by fragmenting projectiles including hollow-point bullets, or with evidence of secondary projectiles or repeated fire.

VITAL STRUCTURES INVOLVED

The vital structures involved in the gunshot wound are usually more important than the caliber or velocity of the projectile with regard to the priorities of treatment and the prognosis.[3] As in any traumatic wound, airway, breathing, and cardiovascular injuries are of immediate importance, whereas musculoskeletal injuries are of secondary consequence. However, synovial and skeletal injuries may significantly affect athletic performance in the horse, and can be life-threatening as well, because of loss of function.

WOUND

The defect caused by the bullet can be classified as nonpenetrating, penetrating, or perforating.[1,8,17] Nonpenetrating wounds can be described as abrasions or injuries affecting the dermis and subcutaneous tissues. Penetrating injuries are those that enter deeper tissues, but do not exit the animal. Because of the elasticity of skin, bullets are often stopped subcutaneously at the end of their wound paths. In this type of wound the kinetic energy of the bullet is fully dissipated in the animal. In perforating bullet wounds, there is an entrance and an exit wound, indicating that the energy was not completely transmitted within the tract. This type of wound tends to be more severe, depending on projectile type and the structures the bullet crosses, because of the amount of kinetic energy required for complete perforation.

FRACTURES

Damage to bony structures is directly related to the energy of the bullet, as well as the type of bone involved. Porous or cancellous bone, such as in the nasal sinuses, shows a circular defect, whereas impact with cortical bone causes spiral or comminuted fractures. As the energy of the projectile increases, so does the degree of comminution.[3] The distinction between extra-articular and intra-articular fractures is important in the classification of bullet injuries because of the risk of joint infection as well as the possibility of joint damage that can affect future athletic performance.

CONTAMINATION

Although contamination of the wound has not been shown to be a significant factor in the human grading scale, this category remains in place because of its clinical relevance.[16] A bullet is not a sterile object, and bacteria can be introduced on the projectile before firing, from objects it encounters in its path, and from the animal's skin.[17] The velocity of the bullet can increase the risk of contamination, because of increased soft tissue damage and necrosis. However, the overall risk of infection is low, unless the bullet has encountered the gastrointestinal tract or structures of the airway. In these cases, the wound should be classified as contaminated, and efforts to remove the bullet should be made.[14]

TREATMENT OF BULLET WOUNDS

The tissues involved are often the most important factor in determining the importance and severity of the wound, rather than the type of bullet and caliber. As with any penetrating trauma, the crushed tissues in the permanent cavity caused by the bullet's path do not survive. Surgical debridement of the damaged tissues depends on depth of the tract and the organs and structures involved. The structures surrounding the bullet's path must also be assessed for viability and potentially debrided because of injury caused by secondary cavitation and shock waves. During the first 3 hours after wounding, the tissues surrounding the primary tract experience a vasoconstrictive phase, affecting color, contractility and consistency of the structures and influencing surgical decision making. After this time, hyperemia and hemorrhage may be noted.[11,14] Therefore, a more conservative approach is required in acute wound management, because of overinterpretation of the severity of the acute injury.

Treatment of bullet wounds centers on reducing contamination introduced by the projectile and from the environment at the entrance and exit wounds. The wound should be left open to allow drainage and further debridement. High-energy wounds are more likely to have not only contamination but more devitalized tissue, which increases the risk of infection. A study on bullet wounds in dogs noted exponential aerobic bacterial growth within 12 hours of wounding, to concentrations greater than 10^5 microorganisms per gram, consistent with tissue levels associated with wound infection.[18] Anaerobes were noted at similar levels in the tissues within 6 hours of the injury. Therefore, systemic broad-spectrum antibiotics that cover aerobic and anaerobic bacteria are indicated, especially if contaminated viscus has been crossed by the bullet's path. It is unlikely that enough lead will leach from a bullet in soft tissues to cause toxicity. Therefore, removal is not indicated for prevention of toxicosis.[19] One exception is lead or copper pellets within synovial structures, which are known to result in a synovitis (**Fig. 4**).[13]

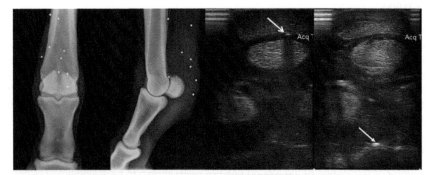

Fig. 4. A 14-year-old American quarter horse presented for a shotgun wound to the right hind fetlock. There are numerous pellets in the soft tissues of the plantar aspect of the limb. Ultrasonography shows a pellet lodged between the superficial and deep digital flexor tendons, proximal to the proximal sesamoid bones (*arrow*, third panel). A second pellet is noted against the plantar third metatarsal bone (*arrow*, fourth panel). The horse was reexamined 2 months later for continued tenosynovitis caused by the intrasynovial pellets (gunshot wound score: LE-S, V-2, W-2, F-0, C-1).

HEAD, NECK, AND SPINE INJURIES

Cerebral penetration by a bullet is often fatal, and in the horse is still an approved method of euthanasia.[20] If the horse survives an accidental gunshot, removal of the projectile is not recommended, and has not been shown to improve the outcome in humans (**Fig. 5**).[21,22] However, if cerebrospinal fluid leakage is noted, it should be addressed.[23] Although surgical approaches to the brain have been described,[24] most equine cranial fractures are medically managed with the aggressive use of antibiotics that penetrate the blood-brain barrier, analgesics, osmotic agents, and anti-inflammatories.[25] Systemic hypotension should be avoided to preserve negative effects on cerebral perfusion pressure, therefore fluid therapy should be provided to maintain euvolemia.[26] For treatment of increased intracranial pressure, mannitol, hypertonic saline, or colloids have been recommended and work best when plasma osmolality is less than 320 mOsm/L.[27] Although mannitol has an antioxidant effect, it may also cause diuresis and acute renal failure, and has been noted to lose its effect with repeated doses. Hypertonic saline may be more effective, with fewer side effects, and possible positive immunomodulatory effects.[28] Neurologic status should be reassessed daily.

In gunshot wounds to the neck, the involvement of large vessels may necessitate emergency ligation, packing, or embolization to prevent exsanguination. Although injury to the trachea and larynx should be assessed with radiographs and endoscopy, conservative management may be considered, and is successful in other species (**Fig. 6**).[29] The airway should be secured if compromised, and a tracheostomy performed if upper airway swelling is severe. For pharyngeal and esophageal wounds, surgical exploration and repair are recommended as soon as the patient is stable because of the higher rate of contamination from these injuries.[23]

Spinal trauma caused by a bullet wound has not been reported at this time in the horse. It can be speculated that most injuries would be severe, and the resulting neurologic deficits would likely be grounds for euthanasia. If a full neurologic examination reveals only mild injury, removal of the bullet fragment is not indicated unless

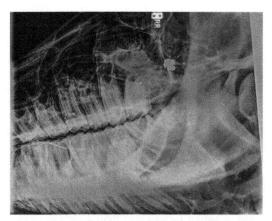

Fig. 5. The skull of a horse with a bullet injury to the frontal and maxillary sinuses caused by a .223 rifle. The bullet penetrated the left caudal maxillary sinus, and lodged in the lateral wall of the right maxillary sinus, noted as a radiolucent density, caudal-dorsal to the last molar. It is possible the ethmoid turbinates were also involved. The bullet was not removed, and the horse survived (gunshot wound score: HE-S, V-2, W-2, EF-1, C-2). (*Courtesy of* Dr Vanessa Cook and Dr Anne Kullman, East Lansing, MI.)

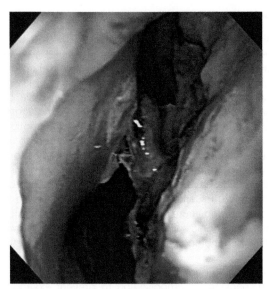

Fig. 6. Endoscopy of the horse in **Fig. 5**. Significant hemorrhage and necrosis of the nasal turbinates was appreciated. On presentation, the horse was hemorrhaging uncontrollably from the nares. A transfusion was required, after bilateral nasal packing and a tracheostomy. (*Courtesy of* Dr Vanessa Cook and Dr Anne Kullman, East Lansing, MI.)

infection results or if the projectile was made of copper, which can have a local necrotic effect.[15,23] Steroids are controversial for any neurologic injury, and no benefit has been observed for treatment of human bullet wounds.[30,31] Other antiinflammatories, including nonsteroidal antiinflammatories, dimethyl sulfoxide, magnesium sulfate, or antioxidants are unproven, but may have a beneficial effect on neurologic outcome.

THORACIC WOUNDS

Cardiac trauma caused by a bullet wound in the horse is usually immediately fatal. Thoracic effusions are more likely to be encountered in surviving horses, including hemothorax and pneumothorax, and can result from the external wound or lacerations of the great vessels, pulmonary parenchyma, or airways.[32] First aid involves sealing the entrance and exit wounds with an airtight dressing, and assessment of airway status and tissue oxygenation. In addition to vital parameters and auscultation, an arterial blood gas analysis or plasma lactate level can be helpful. Once the patient is stable, diagnostics including radiographs and ultrasonography can identify the type and severity of the effusion. If hypoxia or dyspnea are recognized concurrently with a thoracic effusion, thoracocentesis may improve oxygenation. A 24-F chest tube should be placed high in the 13th to 14th rib space for pneumothorax and ventrally at the sixth to eighth rib space for thoracic effusions. If hemorrhage is the cause of the thoracic effusion, fluid resuscitation should be conservative, to maintain a blood pressure of 60 mm Hg, a serum lactate less than 4 mmol/L, blood pH greater than 7.25, and a serum creatinine less than 3 mmol/L. If fluid resuscitation does not improve the horse, or if hemorrhage is thought to be ongoing, a transfusion should be provided. Based on human recommendations, thoracic gunshot wounds in horses may be successfully managed medically with limited debridement and antimicrobial therapy.[33,34]

ABDOMINAL WOUNDS

Nonoperative treatment of abdominal gunshot wounds has increased in popularity in human medicine, based on the high complications rates caused by unnecessary exploratory laparotomies.[15,35,36] Similar recommendations can possibly be proposed for the horse, because of the high risk of postoperative infection, herniation, ileus, and adhesions commonly noted after exploratory laparotomies for colic.[37,38] However, the equine practitioner is limited in the scope of noninvasive diagnostics, including magnetic resonance imaging (MRI) and computed tomography, which are used in human medicine as a substitute for surgery. In horses, abdominal surgery should be recommended based on peritoneal fluid analysis, rectal examination, and ultrasonography. Clinical signs of peritonitis, including serosanguinous or suppurative effusions with degenerative neutrophils, or systemic endotoxemia, indicate the need for surgical intervention (**Fig. 7**).[35,36,39,40] Although the bullet may not be recovered, bowel and organ injury can be addressed primarily. The abdomen can also be thoroughly lavaged for treatment of a septic abdomen and to reduce the risk of adhesions. Antibiotics should be continued for 7 days for prophylaxis after a perforated viscus.[23]

SOFT TISSUE INJURIES AND MUSCULOSKELETAL TRAUMA

Injuries to the skin and skeletal muscle are the most common result of bullet injuries in horses. However, survival rates are excellent, and 87% of horses returned to their previous function in one retrospective study.[5] Radiographs should be obtained, and MRI may be helpful for distal limb injuries. Caution should be taken if the bullet is suspected to be steel (commonly used in birdshot), which can be affected by the magnetic forces.[13] On radiographs, intact shot is more likely to be steel, whereas lead shot easily deforms.

Treatment depends on the severity of the wound. Low-energy wounds are typically not associated with significant damage or infection. Superficial debridement of the wound tract, irrigation, and proper wound dressings suffice. Antibiotic administration is at the discretion of the clinician, and depends on the structures involved. For high-energy wounds, such as shotgun injuries at close range, more extensive debridement is needed. In the acute phase, injured muscle can swell to up to 5 times its normal size,

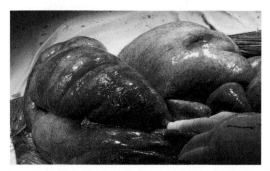

Fig. 7. Intraoperative views of the horse from **Fig. 1**. There are 2 perforations in the ventral colon. The abdominocentesis before surgery noted a total protein of 4.4 g/dL with gross evidence of plant material. The abdomen was lavaged at surgery and for 2 days after surgery. The horse made a full recovery and was discharged 8 days later.

and local edema may cause lactic acidosis and a compartment syndrome that may require fenestration.[2,14] However, the skin and muscle tissue should be allowed to declare themselves, and secondary debridement is often helpful to prevent loss of healthy tissues. Soft tissue wounds should be left open to heal by second intention, because of their contaminated nature.

Synovial structure involvement can be determined by synoviocentesis, and infected structures are best addressed by arthroscopy. Arthrotomy or needle lavage are alternatives, but all should be combined with local antibiotics or regional limb perfusion for improved outcomes. Although the projectile may not be identified, if lead pellets are located within the synovial cavity, they should be removed to prevent synovitis and articular cartilage damage.[13] Fractures are beyond the scope of this article, but should be treated as open, and addressed depending on the possibility of fixation (**Fig. 8**).

LEGAL CONSIDERATIONS

As with any patient, all medical records pertaining to the care and outcome of the patient should be thorough and complete. Local law enforcement or humane officers should also be notified, depending on the laws of the locality. All conversations should be included in the record, and photographic documentation of the wounds should be made. If the projectile is recovered, it should be saved, after gentle cleaning with water and alcohol, in a labeled container. If the horse dies, it is advisable to submit the body to a board-certified pathologist for necropsy.

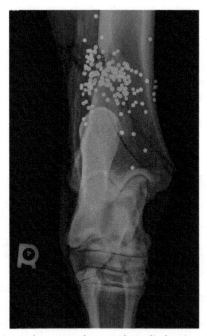

Fig. 8. Close-range (<5 m) gunshot wound to a cadaver limb using 12-gauge steel waterfowl shot. A fracture is noted in the distal tibia, extending into the medial malleolus. Loss of cortical bone is noted on the lateral aspect of the distal diaphysis, where the shot is concentrated (gunshot wound score: HE-2, V-2, W-2, EF-2, C-2).

ACKNOWLEDGMENTS

The authors thank Dr Jack Kottwitz and Dr Robert Cole for assistance with the cadaver radiographs, and Dr Vanessa Cook and Dr Anne Kullman for sharing images of their patients.

REFERENCES

1. Di Maio VJ. Gunshot wounds. In: Practical aspects of firearms, ballistics, and forensic techniques. Boca Raton (FL): CRC Press; 1998.
2. Rozen N, Dudkiewicz I. Wound ballistics and tissue damage. In: Lerner A, Soudry M, editors. Armed conflict injuries to the extremities. Heidelberg: Germany Springer-Verlag; 2011. p. 21–33.
3. Gugala Z, Lindsey RW. Classification of gunshot injuries in civilians. Clin Orthop Relat Res 2003;408:65–81.
4. Hollerman JJ, Fackler ML, Coldwell DM, et al. Gunshot wounds: 1: bullets, ballistics, and mechanisms of injury. Am J Roentgenol 1990;155:685–90.
5. Vatistas NJ, Meagher DM, Gillis CL, et al. Gunshot injuries in horses: 22 cases (1971-1993). J Am Vet Med Assoc 1995;207(9):1198–200.
6. Walker WB, Williams MA, Humberg JM, et al. What is your diagnosis? Radioopaque foreign body (10 × 15 mm) in the pelvic inlet and free peritoneal gas. J Am Vet Med Assoc 1993;202(9):1501–2.
7. Sherman RT, Parrish RA. Management of shotgun injuries: a review of 152 cases. J Trauma 1963;3:76–85.
8. Hopkinson DA, Marshall TK. Firearm injuries. Br J Surg 1967;54:344–53.
9. Volgas DA, Stannard JP, Alonso JE. Ballistics: a primer for the surgeon. Injury 2005;36(3):373–9.
10. Dodd MJ. Terminal ballistics: a text and atlas of gunshot wounds. Boca Raton (FL): CRC Press; 2006. p. 3–124.
11. Alexandropoulou CA, Panagiotopoulos EE. Wound ballistics: analysis of blunt and penetrating trauma mechanisms. Health Sci J 2010;4(4):225–36.
12. Fackler ML. Civilian gunshot wounds and ballistics: dispelling the myths. Emerg Med Clin North Am 1998;16:17–28.
13. Hollerman JJ. Gunshot wounds: 2. Radiology. Am J Roentgenol 1990;155: 691–702.
14. Bartlett CS, Helfet DL, Hausman MR, et al. Ballistics and gunshot wounds: effects on musculoskeletal tissues. J Am Acad Orthop Surg 2000;8:21–36.
15. Lichte P, Oberbeck R, Binnebosel M, et al. A civilian perspective on ballistic trauma and gunshot injuries. Scand J Trauma Resusc Emerg Med 2010. http://dx.doi.org/10.1186/1757-7241-18-35.
16. Brito SA, Gugala Z, Tan A, et al. Statistical validity and clinical merits of a new civilian gunshot injury classification. Clin Orthop Relat Res 2013;471: 3981–7.
17. Mendelson JA. The relationship between mechanisms of wounding and principles of treatment of missile wounds. J Trauma 1991;31:1181–202.
18. Tian HH, Deng GG, Huang MJ, et al. Quantitative bacteriological study of the wound track. J Trauma 1988;28(Suppl):S215–6.
19. Ordog GJ. Lead toxicity secondary to retained missiles. In: Ordog GJ, editor. Management of gunshot wounds. Amsterdam: Elsevier; 1988. p. 405–11.
20. Longair JA, Finley GG, Laniel MA, et al. Guidelines for the euthanasia of domestic animals by firearms. Can Vet J 1991;32:724–6.

21. Hofbauer M, Kdolsky R, Figl M, et al. Predictive factors influencing outcome after gunshot injuries to the head, a retrospective cohort study. J Trauma 2010;69(4): 770–5.

22. Kim TW, Lee JK, Moon KS, et al. Penetrating gunshot injuries to the brain. J Trauma 2007;62:1446–51.

23. Bono CM, Heary RF. Gunshot wounds to the spine. Spine J 2004;4:230–40.

24. Kramer J, Coates JR, Hoffman AG, et al. Preliminary anatomic investigation of three approaches to the equine cranium and brain for limited craniectomy procedures. Vet Surg 2007;36(5):500–8. Available at: http://www.ncbi.nlm.nih.gov/pubmed?term=Frappier%20BL%5BAuthor%5D&cauthor=true&cauthor_uid=17614932.

25. Feary DJ, Magdesian KG, Aleman MA, et al. Traumatic brain injury in horses: 34 cases (1994-2004). J Am Vet Med Assoc 2007;231(2):259–66. Available at: http://www.ncbi.nlm.nih.gov/pubmed?term=Rhodes%20DM%5BAuthor%5D&cauthor=true&cauthor_uid=17630894.

26. Chesnut RM, Marshall LF, Klauber MR, et al. The role of secondary brain injury in determining outcome from severe head injury. J Trauma 1993;34(2):216–22.

27. Adelson PD, Bratton SL, Carney NA, et al. Guidelines for the acute medical management of severe traumatic brain injury in infants, children, and adolescents. Pediatr Crit Care Med 2003;3:S72–5.

28. Kamel H, Navi B, Nakagawa K, et al. Hypertonic saline versus mannitol for the treatment of elevated intracranial pressure: a meta-analysis of randomized clinical trials. Crit Care Med 2011;39(3):554–9.

29. Velmahos GC, Souter I, Degiannis E, et al. Selective surgical management in penetrating neck injuries. Can J Surg 1994;37(6):487–91.

30. Heary RF, Vaccaro AR, Mesa JJ, et al. Steroids and gunshot wounds to the spine. Neurosurgery 1997;41:576–83.

31. Sidhu GS, Ghag A, Prokuski V, et al. Civilian gunshot injuries of the spinal cord: a systematic review of the current literature. Clin Orthop Relat Res 2013;471(12): 3945–55.

32. Hassel DM. Thoracic trauma in horses. Vet Clin North Am Equine Pract 2007; 23(1):67–80.

33. Bastos R, Baisden CE, Harker L, et al. Penetrating thoracic trauma. Semin Thorac Cardiovasc Surg 2008;20(1):19–25. Available at: http://www.ncbi.nlm.nih.gov/pubmed?term=Calhoon%20JH%5BAuthor%5D&cauthor=true&cauthor_uid=18420122.

34. Demetriades D, Velmahos GC. Penetrating injuries of the chest: indications for operation. Scand J Surg 2002;91(1):41–5.

35. Como JJ, Bokhari F, Chiu WC, et al. Practice management guidelines for selective nonoperative management of penetrating abdominal trauma. J Trauma 2010; 68(3):721–33.

36. Inaba K, Demetriades D. The nonoperative management of penetrating abdominal trauma. Adv Surg 2007;41:51–62.

37. Mair TS, Smith LJ. Survival and complication rates in 300 horses undergoing surgical treatment of colic. Part 2: short-term complications. Equine Vet J 2005; 37(4):303–9.

38. Mair TS, Smith LJ. Survival and complication rates in 300 horses undergoing surgical treatment of colic. Part 3: long-term complications and survival. Equine Vet J 2005;37(4):310–4.

39. Biffl WL, Moore EE. Management guidelines for penetrating abdominal trauma. Curr Opin Crit Care 2010;16(6):609–17.

40. Pryor JP, Reilly PM, Dabrowski GP, et al. Nonoperative management of abdominal gunshot wounds. Ann Emerg Med 2004;43(3):344–53.

Infection Control in Equine Critical Care Settings

Brandy A. Burgess, DVM, MSc, PhD[a], Paul S. Morley, DVM, PhD[b],*

KEYWORDS

- Health care–associated infections • Nosocomial infections • Infection control
- Equine

KEY POINTS

- There is a recognizable standard of practice with respect to infection control. Due effort must be given to control and prevention of infectious disease transmission both within a facility and among animal populations: optimal patient care cannot be realized without controlling for health care–associated infections (HCAIs).
- Infection control in the critical care setting is a particular challenge because these patients typically have a greater degree of systemic illness and immune compromise; are more commonly subjected to invasive procedures and placement of indwelling devices; and more frequently receive antimicrobials and gastric protectants, putting them at greater risk for development of HCAIs compared with the general hospital population.
- Every equine critical care unit is distinctive in its physical and operational features and the types of patients that are managed in this hospital area. These unique features necessitate an infection control program be tailored in its finer details to each facility's needs. Designs should be patient centered and present performance guidelines: form should follow function.

IMPORTANCE OF INFECTION CONTROL IN THE CRITICAL CARE SETTING

Optimal patient care cannot be realized without controlling risks for health care–associated infections (HCAIs)[1]: first do no harm. HCAIs result in increased hospitalization duration, increased morbidity and mortality among affected patients, and can greatly increase the cost of care.[2] In 2002, there were an estimated 4.5 HCAIs per 100 human hospital admissions, with an estimated 5.8% of deaths associated with HCAIs in the United States,[3] which is more than are reported for notifiable diseases. These deaths are therefore among the top 10 causes of human deaths reported in the United States.[3]

Critical care patients are a unique part of hospital populations in both human and veterinary hospitals. In general, compared with patient groups that are less sick,

[a] Department of Population Health Sciences, Virginia-Maryland Regional College of Veterinary Medicine, Virginia Tech, 100 Sandy Hall, MC 0395, Blacksburg, VA 24061-0395, USA; [b] Department of Clinical Sciences, James L. Voss Veterinary Teaching Hospital, Colorado State University, 1678 Campus Delivery, Fort Collins, CO 80526, USA
* Corresponding author.
E-mail address: paul.morley@colostate.edu

Vet Clin Equine 30 (2014) 467–474
http://dx.doi.org/10.1016/j.cveq.2014.04.009
0749-0739/14/$ – see front matter © 2014 Elsevier Inc. All rights reserved.
vetequine.theclinics.com

critical care patients have more systemic illness, a greater degree of immune compromise, are more commonly subjected to invasive procedures and placement of indwelling devices, and more commonly receive antimicrobials and gastric protectants. All of these factors place them at greater risk for development of HCAIs compared with the general hospital population. As a result, it was recently estimated that approximately 30% of adult intensive care patients in developed countries experience an HCAI during hospitalization, which is approximately a 10 times greater risk for HCAI than is seen among noncritical patients in human hospitals.[4]

Although similar data in veterinary medicine are lacking, the occurrence of HCAIs is common among accredited veterinary teaching hospitals (VTHs) and there are several publications documenting large outbreaks of HCAIs associated with a variety of contagious agents. In a survey regarding infection control programs at these hospitals, 82% reported outbreaks of HCAIs in the preceding 5 years, with 58% resulting in restrictions to patient admission and 32% reporting facility closure to aid mitigation efforts.[5] In adult horses admitted for gastrointestinal disorders, approximately 20% experienced an HCAI during hospitalization based on syndromic surveillance from 5 participating VTHs in a 6-week period.[6] Despite the recognized occurrence of outbreaks, the sporadic occurrence of HCAIs is poorly understood. Further, because most veterinary hospitals do not use a systematic approach for documenting or investigating the occurrence of HCAIs, practices used for preventing infections are almost entirely based on empiric assumptions.

Regardless of the paucity of evidence on which to base veterinary infection control practices, there is a clear risk to veterinary patients and personnel working with these animals. There are equally clear ethical and legal obligations for veterinarians to make a concerted effort to address these issues. Stated another way, there is a recognizable standard of practice with respect to infection control and due effort must be given to control and prevention of infectious disease transmission both within a facility and among animal populations: it is possible to do too little.[7]

GENERAL INFECTION CONTROL CONCEPTS

Infection control is embodied by all efforts used to prevent the introduction and contain the spread of contagious pathogens within a facility or population. Overarching goals of an infection control program (ICP) are to eliminate sources of potentially pathogenic microorganisms and to break transmission cycles. In veterinary hospital settings, this is a challenge because clinicians are purposefully caring for patients with infectious diseases, and also generally caring for patients whose resistance to disease is compromised (especially those patients managed in the critical care unit [CCU]) and doing so in an environment that congregates animals from many different farms that are likely to be harboring an infectious agent.

There are several types of preventive measures that can be used to decrease infectious disease transmission risk, including environmental and personal hygiene and managing patient contacts. Specific measures to be used include early detection of high-risk patients, rigorous hand hygiene and contact precautions (ie, barrier nursing precautions), patient cohorting, movement restriction (including patient isolation), and regular environmental sanitation and monitoring (when information regarding contamination with specific pathogens is used to guide mitigation efforts). Every equine hospital is distinctive in physical and operational features, as well as in the different types of patients that are managed. These unique features necessitate an ICP being tailored in its details to each facility's needs. All ICPs that should be incorporated address these common infection control principles. There are general systematic approaches, such as the Hazard Analysis and Critical Control Point (HACCP) system, which have previously been described to facilitate program development.[8] Although the choice of policies governing an ICP vary by facility, it is important that they are designed with all animals in mind, not just those suspected of harboring an infectious disease.

Many of the practices used in veterinary infection control have not been scientifically evaluated; however, clinicians can draw from knowledge gained from infection control strategies applied in human health care. Design of an equine CCU is one such area. The overarching goal is to minimize the introduction, spread, and persistence of potential pathogens and to create an environment that facilitates rigorous cleaning and disinfection of any potentially contaminated surface. In general, there needs to be sufficient space to facilitate patient management, numerous hand hygiene stations, isolation facilities with appropriate ventilation, and sufficient storage space to house specialized equipment.[9,10] Designs should be patient centered and present guidelines that accommodate the necessary functions that are to be performed in the area (ie, performance guidelines): form should follow function.[11] In an equine CCU, this depends on the types of cases managed in this area, but may include adequate space for managing the adult postoperative colic, mare-foal pairs, critically ill foals that may need sophisticated life support (eg, mechanical ventilation), and the critically ill patients whose disease is directly related to contagious diseases such as those caused by *Salmonella* or equine herpesvirus-1. Consideration should also be given to creating separate areas to care for adult and neonatal critical care patients. It is important when extrapolating from human health care to keep in mind that the level of environmental contamination is typically much greater in veterinary hospitals than in human health care facilities and that veterinary patients defecate in the locale in which they are housed, creating unique challenges in the prevention of HCAIs.

CHALLENGES OF INFECTION CONTROL IN THE CRITICAL CARE SETTING

The combination of the need for sophisticated intensive care, the difficulties associated with managing patients with challenges regarding physical needs (eg, adult horses with neurologic disease), and the need to prevent contact and aerosol transmission of highly contagious agents presents extreme challenges in the design and management of equine intensive care units. Specific consideration should be given to infection control practices implemented in an equine CCU, in addition to those that might be used in other areas. Not only is this unit likely to house patients harboring potential pathogens but it is also where the most compromised patients are managed, including patients that are extremely susceptible to developing HCAIs. A painful horse is one that wants to lie down and roll and, given that such animals are housed where they defecate and urinate, this creates ample opportunity to contaminate catheter sites (including intravenous, epidural, and urinary catheters) and surgical wounds with potential pathogens residing in the hospital environment.

Risks Associated with Caretaker-Patient Contacts

In general, because of the need for intensive monitoring and invasive interventions, critically ill patients require more frequent contact with health care providers, creating greater opportunity for infectious disease transmission. Thus all caretakers working in critical care settings should take extra precautions when managing these patients. These actions may include increased attention to hand hygiene, use of gloves when managing catheters, use of barrier nursing precautions (ie, a barrier gown, gloves, and footwear hygiene) when managing a colic or critical neonate, and use of separate cleaning equipment.

Risks Associated with Intravenous Catheterization

Intravenous catheters create a portal of entry for potential pathogens. Thus catheter sites should be aseptically prepared and checked daily for thrombophlebitis (ie, pain, swelling, redness, and discharge).[12] It is also important to effectively immobilize catheters so as to reduce the potential for irritation and infections at the site of placement. If inflammation or signs of infection are noted, the catheter should be removed aseptically and a new one placed at an alternative site, saving the removed catheter tip for bacterial culture.

Catheter infections are commonly associated with the introduction of bacteria through the catheter hub; catheter hub colonization accounts for an estimated 70% of catheter-related sepsis in human patients receiving total parenteral nutrition.[13] Therefore, it is recommended that the catheter hub be cleaned with alcohol or iodine before injecting with a sterile needle and syringe.[12] Bacteria colonizing catheter tips among equids are most commonly resident skin flora, including *Staphylococcus*, *Corynebacterium*, *Bacillus*, *Enterobacter*, and *Pseudomonas* spp.[12]

Catheter site inflammation has been reported to occur, on average, in 8.8% of equine admissions to a CCU for gastrointestinal disease[6] and approximately 18% (7 of 38) of postoperative colics with catheters in place for an average of 3.5 days.[14] Catheter-related complications (eg, thrombosis, phlebitis) are reported to be higher in foals receiving parenteral nutrition; up to 15% with approximately one-half having culture-positive catheter tips.[15,16]

Special Considerations When Managing Critically Ill Foals

Foals that are critically ill present additional challenges in that they are commonly severely immunocompromised, unable to stand, semiconscious or comatose, and require continuous monitoring. All of these conditions necessitate rigorous attention to hygiene. Not only are precautions needed to limit spread of potential pathogens from a sick foal to the other patients but it is important to protect these patients from exposure to potentially harmful pathogens residing in the hospital environment. Contaminated environmental surfaces can play an important role in the transmission of infectious agents.[17,18] Every effort should be made to use barrier nursing techniques including gowns, gloves, and footwear hygiene (eg, shoe covers, disinfectant mats), and to practice rigorous hand hygiene (washing hands or using an alcohol-based hand sanitizer) before and after every person comes in contact with the foal.

RISKS ASSOCIATED WITH MANAGING CRITICAL CARE PATIENTS
What Are the Risks?

In veterinary medicine, understanding of the risks associated with developing HCAIs is limited. Although there have been studies evaluating factors associated with events such as surgical site infections in postoperative colics and catheter site–associated thrombophlebitis, only a single study has more generally broached the topic of how commonly HCAIs occur in equine hospitals. Among horses hospitalized in CCUs for gastrointestinal disorders, 19.7% (95% confidence interval [CI], 14.5, 26.7) experienced at least one HCAI based on syndromic surveillance.[6] The most common HCAIs identified through syndromic surveillance were surgical site inflammation (12.9%) and intravenous catheter site inflammation (8.8%). Among the top 5 short-term complications (ie, from anesthesia recovery to hospital discharge) reported for horses having a single laparotomy were incisional drainage or infection and jugular thrombophlebitis. One study reported incisional infections in almost one-third (28.9%) and jugular catheter–related infections in approximately 8%.[19] Almost half of horses (43%) experienced incisional infections in another study.[20] If a horse required a second laparotomy, the odds of developing incisional drainage or infection increased by 2 times (odds ratio [OR], 2.15; 95% CI, 0.86, 5.23).[19] In addition, those experiencing wound complications and repeat laparotomy were more likely to develop a ventral hernia 2 to 3 months after hospital discharge.[21] Minimizing the potential for developing a surgical site infection is critical to decreasing morbidity and having a successful patient outcome.

Many factors that occur before or during surgery have significant impact on infection risks (eg, surgery duration, perioperative antimicrobial therapy, anesthesia and ventilation protocols), but postoperative care can also significantly influence the risk for HCAIs.[20,22] Although placing a stent bandage over a surgical incision has produced disparate results, some researchers finding increased odds of wound complications (OR, 19.16; 95% CI, 5.37, 102.54) and others finding a reduction (OR, 0.10; 95% CI, 0.02, 0.50), research suggests that placing a wound cover during anesthesia recovery reduces the odds of experiencing wound complications, which may reflect less contamination and tissue trauma during surgery or better wound management after surgery.[19,23] This finding implies that strategies to prevent HCAIs should be an integral part of patient management at the initiation of treatment and throughout hospitalization.

Specific Agents of Concern

There are many infections agents that may be considered when implementing infection control in a critical care setting but there are some that warrant specific mention, including *Clostridium difficile*, rotavirus, and *Salmonella enterica*.

C difficile can frequently be found in the gastrointestinal flora of healthy horses and foals. However, enteric disease can develop when toxigenic strains are present and disturbance of the normal gastrointestinal flora allows clostridial organisms to occupy a larger niche in the microbiome, such as during the stress of hospitalization, as a result of gastrointestinal disease, or with antimicrobial therapy.[24,25] Clostridial spores are resistant to disinfection and can be detected throughout the large animal clinical environment despite standard environmental measures being used.[26] Because this pathogen is transmitted by the fecal-oral route, rigorous environmental and hand hygiene is imperative to disrupting the transmission cycle and eliminating the environment as a reservoir for this potential pathogen.

Rotaviruses are a common cause of diarrhea in foals, being detected in 20% to 35% of foals with gastrointestinal disease, and are considered to be ubiquitous in the equine population.[27,28] They are highly contagious, environmentally persistent, and transmitted by the fecal-oral route. Therefore, rigorous hand and environmental hygiene is important in disrupting the transmission cycle and eliminating environmental reservoirs. Although there are vaccines available, current research on efficacy remains equivocal.[29]

S enterica is a common cause of epidemics of HCAIs.[5] In the course of epidemic disease, horses with severe disease (eg, colic or undergoing abdominal surgery) are frequently identified as shedding *Salmonella* and likely contribute to ongoing environmental contamination and transmission among hospitalized patients.[30–33] Recovery of genetically related *Salmonella* Infantis isolates during routine surveillance of patients and the hospital environment over an extended period of time suggests environmental persistence and ongoing transmission despite implementation of a rigorous ICP, emphasizing the importance of eliminating reservoirs for infection within the hospital environment.[34]

Eliminating Environmental Persistence of Potential Pathogens

In human health care facilities, the environment near where patients positive to methicillin-resistant *Staphylococcus aureus* (MRSA) are managed can remain contaminated despite rigorous environmental hygiene, which shows the important role the environment can play in ongoing transmission of potential pathogens.[35] Proper use of cleaning and disinfection (a multistep process involving the removal of visible debris, scrubbing with a detergent, followed by rinsing and application of an appropriate disinfectant at the correct dilution and contact time) are fundamental to eliminating sources of infectious agents and breaking the cycle of transmission. Although rigorous cleaning alone can reduce the bacterial load on a concrete surface by 90%, applying an appropriate disinfectant after cleaning can reduce this by an additional 6%.[36] Cleaning protocols should be clearly delineated and surveillance should be conducted to ensure compliance and that protocols remain effective in the ever-changing environment of the veterinary hospital.[7]

SUMMARY

HCAIs are those that were not present or incubating when the patient was admitted to the hospital. In general, the potential for infections to be HCAIs should be suspected if they develop after 48 to 72 hours of hospitalization (however, this varies by microorganism and with the degree of patient compromise).[37] Advances in human health care have shown the efficacy of implementing a comprehensive ICP (ie, using trained personnel, conducting surveillance activity, and reporting back to stakeholders) for reducing the occurrence of HCAIs.[38] Although it is reasonable to assume the likelihood of a reduced HCAI rate in veterinary hospitals implementing an effective ICP, equivalent data are lacking in veterinary medicine. So how do clinicians assess the effectiveness of prevention efforts used in the practice of veterinary medicine? They must first understand the baseline risk to their patients of important health care–associated outcomes. A study of equine patients receiving critical care found that at least one nosocomial event (ie, surgical site inflammation, intravenous catheter site inflammation, gastrointestinal disorders, fever of unknown origin, acute respiratory disorders, sepsis, or urinary tract inflammation) occurred in an estimated 19.7% of admissions, which is equivalent to 3.9 cases per 100 hospitalization days.[6] This finding represents a starting place to help determine whether a prevention measure affects the occurrence of undesirable health care–associated outcomes and ultimately an avenue to acquire evidence on which to base infection control practices in veterinary medicine.

REFERENCES

1. Morley PS. Evidence-based infection control in clinical practice: if you buy clothes for the emperor, will he wear them? J Vet Intern Med 2013;27(3):430–8.
2. Calfee DP. Crisis in hospital-acquired, healthcare-associated infections. Annu Rev Med 2012;63:359–71.
3. Klevens RM, Edwards JR, Richards CL, et al. Estimating health care-associated infections and deaths in U.S. hospitals, 2002. Public Health Rep 2007;122(2): 160–6.
4. Vincent JL. Nosocomial infections in adult intensive-care units. Lancet 2003; 361(9374):2068–77.
5. Benedict KM, Morley PS, Van Metre DC. Characteristics of biosecurity and infection control programs at veterinary teaching hospitals. J Am Vet Med Assoc 2008; 233(5):767–73.
6. Ruple-Czerniak AA, Aceto HW, Bender JB, et al. Syndromic surveillance for evaluating the occurrence of healthcare-associated infections in equine hospitals. Equine Vet J 2013. http://dx.doi.org/10.1111/evj.12190.

7. Morley PS, Anderson ME, Burgess BA, et al. Report of the third Havemeyer work-shop on infection control in equine populations. Equine Vet J 2012;45:131–6.
8. Morley PS. Biosecurity of veterinary practices. Vet Clin North Am Food Anim Pract 2002;18(1):133–55, vii.
9. O'Connell NH, Humphreys H. Intensive care unit design and environmental factors in the acquisition of infection. J Hosp Infect 2000;45(4):255–62.
10. Dettenkofer M, Seegers S, Antes G, et al. Does the architecture of hospital facilities influence nosocomial infection rates? A systematic review. Infect Control Hosp Epidemiol 2004;25(1):21–5.
11. Thompson DR, Hamilton DK, Cadenhead CD, et al. Guidelines for intensive care unit design. Crit Care Med 2012;40(5):1586–600.
12. Tan RH, Dart AJ, Dowling BA. Catheters: a review of the selection, utilisation and complications of catheters for peripheral venous access. Aust Vet J 2003;81(3): 136–9.
13. Linares J, Sitges-Serra A, Garau J, et al. Pathogenesis of catheter sepsis: a prospective study with quantitative and semiquantitative cultures of catheter hub and segments. J Clin Microbiol 1985;21(3):357–60.
14. Lankveld DP, Ensink JM, van Dijk P, et al. Factors influencing the occurrence of thrombophlebitis after post-surgical long-term intravenous catheterization of colic horses: a study of 38 cases. J Vet Med A Physiol Pathol Clin Med 2001;48(9): 545–52.
15. Krause JB, McKenzie HC. Parenteral nutrition in foals: a retrospective study of 45 cases (2000–2004). Equine Vet J 2007;39(1):74–8.
16. Myers CJ, Magdesian KG, Kass PH, et al. Parenteral nutrition in neonatal foals: clinical description, complications and outcome in 53 foals (1995-2005). Vet J 2009;181(2):137–44.
17. Dancer SJ. Mopping up hospital infection. J Hosp Infect 1999;43(2):85–100.
18. Carling PC, Bartley JM. Evaluating hygienic cleaning in health care settings: what you do not know can harm your patients. Am J Infect Control 2010;38(5): S41–50.
19. Mair TS, Smith LJ. Survival and complication rates in 300 horses undergoing surgical treatment of colic. Part 2: short-term complications. Equine Vet J 2005; 37(4):303–9.
20. Freeman KD, Southwood LL, Lane J, et al. Post operative infection, pyrexia and perioperative antimicrobial drug use in surgical colic patients. Equine Vet J 2012; 44(4):476–81.
21. Mair TS, Smith LJ. Survival and complication rates in 300 horses undergoing surgical treatment of colic. Part 3: long-term complications and survival. Equine Vet J 2005;37(4):310–4.
22. Costa-Farre C, Prades M, Ribera T, et al. Does intraoperative low arterial partial pressure of oxygen increase the risk of surgical site infection following emergency exploratory laparotomy in horses? Vet J 2014. http://dx.doi.org/10.1016/j.tvjl.2014.01.029.
23. Tnibar A, Grubbe Lin K, Thuroe Nielsen K, et al. Effect of a stent bandage on the likelihood of incisional infection following exploratory coeliotomy for colic in horses: a comparative retrospective study. Equine Vet J 2013;45(5):564–9.
24. Diab SS, Songer G, Uzal FA. *Clostridium difficile* infection in horses: a review. Vet Microbiol 2013;167(1–2):42–9.
25. Baverud V, Gustafsson A, Franklin A, et al. *Clostridium difficile*: prevalence in horses and environment, and antimicrobial susceptibility. Equine Vet J 2003; 35(5):465–71.

26. Weese JS, Staempfli HR, Prescott JF. Isolation of environmental *Clostridium difficile* from a veterinary teaching hospital. J Vet Diagn Invest 2000;12(5):449–52.

27. Slovis NM, Elam J, Estrada M, et al. Infectious agents associated with diarrhoea in neonatal foals in central Kentucky: a comprehensive molecular study. Equine Vet J 2014;46:311–6.

28. Frederick JS, Giguere S, Sanchez LC. Infectious agents detected in the feces of diarrheic foals: a retrospective study of 233 cases (2003-2008). J Vet Intern Med 2009;23(6):254–60.

29. Bailey KE, Gilkerson JR, Browning GF. Equine rotaviruses–current understanding and continuing challenges. Vet Microbiol 2013;167(1–2):135–44.

30. Tillotson K, Savage CJ, Salman MD, et al. Outbreak of *Salmonella* Infantis infection in a large animal veterinary teaching hospital. J Am Vet Med Assoc 1997; 211(12):1554–7.

31. House JK, Mainar-Jaime RC, Smith BP, et al. Risk factors for nosocomial *Salmonella* infection among hospitalized horses. J Am Vet Med Assoc 1999;214(10): 1511–6.

32. Ekiri AB, MacKay RJ, Gaskin JM, et al. Epidemiologic analysis of nosocomial *Salmonella* infections in hospitalized horses. J Am Vet Med Assoc 2009;234(1): 108–19.

33. Hird DW, Pappaioanou M, Smith BP. Case-control study of risk factors associated with isolation of *Salmonella* Saintpaul in hospitalized horses. Am J Epidemiol 1984;120(6):852–64.

34. Dunowska M, Morley PS, Traub-Dargatz JL, et al. Comparison of *Salmonella enterica* serotype Infantis isolates from a veterinary teaching hospital. J Appl Microbiol 2007;102(6):1527–36.

35. Blythe D, Keenlyside D, Dawson SJ, et al. Environmental contamination due to methicillin-resistant *Staphylococcus aureus* (MRSA). J Hosp Infect 1998;38(1): 67–9.

36. Dwyer RM. Environmental disinfection to control equine infectious diseases. Vet Clin North Am Equine Pract 2004;20(3):531–42.

37. Garner JS, Jarvis WR, Emori TG, et al. CDC definitions for nosocomial infections, 1988. Am J Infect Control 1988;16(3):128–40.

38. Haley RW, Culver DH, White JW, et al. The efficacy of infection surveillance and control programs in preventing nosocomial infections in US hospitals. Am J Epidemiol 1985;121(2):182–205.

Index

Note: Page numbers of article titles are in **boldface** type.

Vet Clin Equine 30 (2014) 475–487
http://dx.doi.org/10.1016/S0749-0739(14)00045-5
0749-0739/14/$ – see front matter © 2014 Elsevier Inc. All rights reserved.

vetequine.theclinics.com

Moving?

Make sure your subscription moves with you!

To notify us of your new address, find your **Clinics Account Number** (located on your mailing label above your name), and contact customer service at:

Email: journalscustomerservice-usa@elsevier.com

800-654-2452 (subscribers in the U.S. & Canada)
314-447-8871 (subscribers outside of the U.S. & Canada)

Fax number: 314-447-8029

Elsevier Health Sciences Division
Subscription Customer Service
3251 Riverport Lane
Maryland Heights, MO 63043

*To ensure uninterrupted delivery of your subscription, please notify us at least 4 weeks in advance of move.

Printed and bound by CPI Group (UK) Ltd, Croydon, CR0 4YY

03/10/2024

01040487-0003